EXPANSIONAL

BALANCE

EXPANSIONAL
BALANCE

A HOLISTIC EXERCISE APPROACH
TO BETTER HEALTH AND FITNESS

BRIAN DOUGAN

Cover and layout design by G Sharp Design, LLC.
www.gsharpmajor.com

ISBN 979-8-9888010-2-3 (paperback)
ISBN 979-8-9888010-1-6 (hardcover)
ISBN 979-8-9888010-0-9 (ebook)
Library of Congress Control Number: 2023913859

PREFACE

I have been working in the holistic health industry since 1989, when I started as a massage therapist. I studied at the international Professional School of Bodywork (IPSB) in San Diego, California, and became a Holistic Health Practitioner (HHP) in 1991. I've also been regularly working out at fitness centers my entire adult life.

My experience in the holistic health and fitness worlds over the years has given me some unique insights. Both the holistic health industry and the fitness industry purport to benefit your health and overall well-being. But they both miss an opportunity to help you do that effectively.

Holistic health practices typically focus on freeing blocked energy and balancing that energy in the body and mind to enhance your health and well-being. However, they tend to lack vigorous exercise regimens that will build strength and endurance for physical fitness. Although strength building via resistance exercises is part of the holistic health paradigm, I've found it's not practiced or encouraged much.

Meanwhile, the fitness industry emphasizes building strength and endurance through vigorous, regimental training with the goal of maximizing performance. But it lacks a focus on building flexibility, balanced movement, and greater body awareness to enhance your health.

This led me to wonder: Why not combine the best aspects of both industries—the fitness industry's "regimental exercise for maximizing performance" and the holistic health world's "balancing mind and body to enhance health and well-being"? Bridging the two paradigms would give us a "regimental holistic program to enhance health and fitness."[1]

In this book, I attempt to provide that bridge. I'm going to give specific examples of exercise routines—ones I've been doing myself for decades—along with explanations of how each exercise contributes to building and maintaining flexibility, balanced movement, and greater body awareness, along with strength and endurance. The outcome? *A higher quality of life.*

This book is not just a "how-to" guide for these exercises. ***Instead, it explains why each exercise is important, what the intent of each exercise is, and how it relates to a holistic approach to health and fitness.*** It assumes a basic familiarity with the exercises in question, as well as with basic anatomy and the proper use of exercise equipment. Beyond that, you just need to bring your curiosity and desire to improve your health and fitness for the rest of your life!

---

1 In this context, "health" is defined as a lack of disease and the proper functioning of all the body's systems, and "fitness" as the capacity to do physical work.

TABLE OF CONTENTS

TABLE OF TABLES

TABLE OF FIGURES

INTRODUCTION

Are you looking for a results-based fitness regimen that allows you to measure and achieve your fitness goals? Are you training to maximize your performance to compete with others? If you answered yes to either question, put this book down and walk away, because it's not for you.

But if you're looking for better overall health and functionality, fewer aches and pains, improved mental alertness, greater ease in daily physical activities, and improved quality of life—for the rest of your life—then this book is for you.

In this book I take a holistic approach to health and fitness. What do I mean by that? Holistic health considers many aspects of wellness. It includes being aware of the relationship between the physical, mental, and spiritual aspects of your health. It means being an active participant in your health decisions and healing processes, including conventional and alternative health modalities.

Holistic health is associated with types of modalities that are derived from ancient healing traditions such as massage, acupuncture, yoga, and energy therapies, to name a few. Holistic approaches are also associated with the use of whole foods, herbs, supplements, teas, homeopathic remedies, and essential oils, to list some examples. Activities that most people associate with the word "holistic" can include drumming, prayer, meditation, dancing, singing, chanting, and mindfulness. Moreover, most holistic health practices are used in combination with each other to provide an integrated approach to health.

A holistic approach means understanding that your physical and emotional health are intertwined. This is known as the mind–body connection. Our chemistry and biology impact our mood and emotions, as well as thoughts and beliefs. If you've ever felt your stomach tighten up when you were anxious, you've experienced the mind–body connection. The basic exercises in this book will help you gain a greater awareness of that connection.

The exercises in this book draw on concepts from a holistic modality called Structural Integration (SI). The intent of SI is to reorganize the body into a neutral, more efficient alignment. SI is done by a practitioner applying pressure to hold tissue in place while asking for movement across a joint—engaging only muscles that are intended for that movement. The pressure from the practitioner's hands releases the surrounding fascia, and movement across the joint becomes easier. If there are any aberrant holding patterns or compensatory muscles continue to engage while pressure is applied to those muscles, then the sensation may be painful to the client. As a result of the session, the client will find movement easier and become more aware of aberrant holding patterns.

Through my experience studying, teaching, and practicing SI for many decades, I've learned to apply the concepts of SI to my exercise regimen—particularly the concept of *expansional balance*, which I explain in the next section.

This book is a guide to achieving the same outcomes you would in a hands-on session with an SI practitioner. Doing these exercises, you'll find the outcome can be enlightening as you release painful and stressful patterns of tension, gain ease of movement and posture, and experience a sense of greater possibilities for using and experiencing your body.

Good Health and Fitness at Any Age

The exercises in this book are a means to a higher quality of life. Unless you have a severe medical condition preventing you from working out, there is no reason, regardless of age, you can't maintain a healthy level of strength, endurance, and flexibility even if you're just beginning to exercise after decades of neglect.

When one's body has an ache or pain that causes them to move with an aberrant gait (such as a limp, or with the back bent) the knee-jerk response I often hear (even from myself) is, "I'm getting too old." Then when the ache or pain clears up and walking becomes normal again, we think nothing of it.

Well, there is a profound lesson to be learned from that experience, one most people overlook. *You don't have to feel you're getting old as long as you keep the aches and pains away!* The exercises in this book will help you do just that.

Many people tell me, "I'm old, and because of that I simply can't do the things I used to do." There is little truth to this argument. The real reason most older people can't do the things they used to is because they haven't been *exercising* the way they used to—sometimes for decades. Exercise is the key to a healthy life. If you don't exercise, your body will become weak, sluggish and stiff, and your quality of life will decline.

When movement becomes painful and our quality of life diminishes, we often appeal to the "experts" to alleviate our ailments. Unfortunately, the experts all too often provide only short-term relief that doesn't solve the underlying issues: Swallow a pill for this ailment, take this prescription to mask your pain, or receive a shot that will lessen the discomfort.

The truth is that you are your own best expert at creating a long and healthy life! A little-known secret you may not be aware of is that the human body has a surprisingly high degree of plasticity—you can continue to mold it as you age. You can become better and stronger with more vitality. The answer is exercise! You're in charge, and you can make it happen.

Exercising vs. Training

Before we start exploring the concept of expansional balance, it's important to understand the distinction between exercising and training—and why this book is based on the former and not the latter.

Training is conditioning the body to excel at a specific endeavor, like running a marathon or weightlifting, to compete with others. It is a chance to show off your physical prowess to others and potentially win a trophy to validate your sacrifices and sweat over the months (or years) of training. Exercising, on the other hand, is to exert yourself physically in ways you wouldn't normally do on a day-to-day basis. The intent of exercising, as opposed to training, is to maintain a level of health that prevents the body from becoming weak, sluggish, and stiff.

This book is not about training your body toward maximizing your physical capabilities to compete with others. Although many people find such an approach fulfilling, it can sometimes lead them to build their personal identity around how well they compete, instead of how their training affects their quality of life. Instead, this book is focused on exercises that will help move you toward a higher quality of life. My aim is to give you the tools you need to feel strong, energetic, mentally alert, and free of aches and pains for the rest of your life.

CHAPTER 1

EXPANSIONAL BALANCE: GRAVITY AS A SOURCE OF HEALTH

How can gravity be a source of health? It may surprise you to learn that our reaction to the force of gravity is what allows the body to feel light and movements to feel effortless. Here's how that works.

Our bodies respond to the force of gravity by expanding outward from the contact surface (usually the ground). This reaction force is then distributed (ideally) equally in all directions. For example, in standing, the feet push into the ground in an equal and opposite reaction to gravity. This allows the skeleton to interact with its fascial struts to unfold outward and upward, letting the head rise easily and creating a vertical (up and down) polarity through the body. This vertical polarity is the first component of "expansional balance" the body achieves in response to gravity.

The second component is horizontal polarity. A key example of horizontal polarity occurs in the movement of the elbows, as they, like the knees for the pelvis, initiate the movement of the limbs out from the spine. The elbows extend from the spine through the shoulder girdle, the arms continue to extend through the center of each joint of the wrists and hands and as far as our fingers can imagine.[2] The outward extension of the arms allows the head to extend further upward. This outward extension, or horizontal polarity, further reinforces expansional balance in the body.

Therefore, gravity is a source of energy we can use to achieve ease and lightness in the body. As the reaction force to gravity comes through the feet, it is transferred to the waist and extends up the torso and out through the arms, neck, and head. The expansion of the body is stabilized by the deep muscles of the core as it passes through the joints of the limbs and beyond the hands and feet.

Gaining and maintaining a sense of expansional balance—the feeling that the body is allowed to extend effortlessly in all directions, one segment upon another—is one of the main goals of the exercises in this book. Let's now explore the concept of expansional balance in more detail, so you can get the maximum benefit out of these exercises.

---

2 If the feet and hands are contracted, then the entire limb is impacted all the way back to the core. It's as if the hands and feet must extend and contact the outside world for the limbs to extend out from the core. The feet are on the ground, thus limiting the movement of the legs. But the hands don't have the same limitation. So, they reach out as far as we can "imagine," ensuring the arms don't become shortened or twisted.

Expansional Balance: The Concept

Moving with expansional balance is an act of moving with no resistance in the joints. When we stand and walk in gravity, the reaction force of the ground wants to be distributed throughout our bodies in all directions. For simplicity, I'll discuss how expansional balance is achieved in just the vertical and horizontal directions. Also, I'll touch on how to align the torso so the reaction force of gravity can move freely upward and be distributed evenly through the legs, torso, shoulders, and up through the head.

Vertical Polarity

Pelvic extension begins the vertical polarity. The lifting of the spine is created when the rear of the pelvis turns downward. This downward turn of the pelvis causes a downward thrust of the feet into the ground. The downward thrust of the feet then causes an upward thrust of the spine, which allows the body's expansional balance for the vertical polarity.

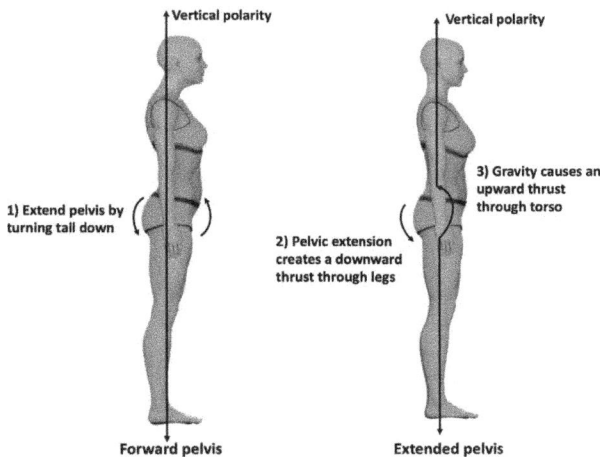

Figure 1: Vertical Polarity

Horizontal Polarity

Arms are much lighter than legs. This is because they are designed to extend outward rather than stabilize the upper body. The arms extend horizontally so the shoulder girdle can balance and allow the head and neck to extend. The extension of the elbows begins the horizontal polarity, defining the sides of the body. The elbows extend from the spine *through* the shoulder girdle, not *from* the shoulder girdle.[3]

Three Rings of the Torso

The torso must be balanced around the center of gravity if the energy from gravity is to pass freely through the body and to the head. The torso consists of three areas or "rings" that shape our core. The three rings are the pelvic ring, diaphragm ring, and shoulder ring. The vertical polarity must pass unimpeded through these three rings to achieve expansional balance.

The first is the pelvic ring, which is balanced and stabilized on the hips. During pelvic extension, the pelvic ring is balanced, with the perineum (the tissue between the thighs that makes up the bottom of the pelvic cavity) at the center of that balance.

The second ring is the diaphragm ring. The vertical polarity moves upward through the balanced pelvic ring, which was established by the downward thrust of the legs. The diaphragm ring comes into a parallel relationship with the pelvic ring, balancing the lumbar area of the spine.

---

3 I'm emphasizing the point of origin of horizontal polarity. When horizontal polarity is initiated by the elbows, then that will cause the arms to swing when walking. A lot of people (especially men), tend to use their shoulders or lean with their shoulders in the direction they're moving. This causes the horizontal polarity to become stuck in their shoulder girdle. Their arms don't swing anymore. The horizontal polarity begins from the spine and passes unimpeded through the shoulder.

The third ring is the shoulder ring. The balanced diaphragm ring becomes the foundation for the shoulder ring. Only by coming into a parallel relationship with the diaphragm ring can the shoulder ring find balance, allowing both the neck and head to rise, and releasing the horizontal polarity. In this way, the shoulder ring acts as a floating intermediary between the vertical and horizontal polarities.

Neck and Head

If there is balance among all three rings of the torso, then the neck and head will naturally find balance. The rising of the head from the neck will feel effortless. In fact, the head just needs to find balance on the atlas joint (the hinge that allows the head to nod). The neck will be balanced from front and back, between the shoulders and down into the upper chest.

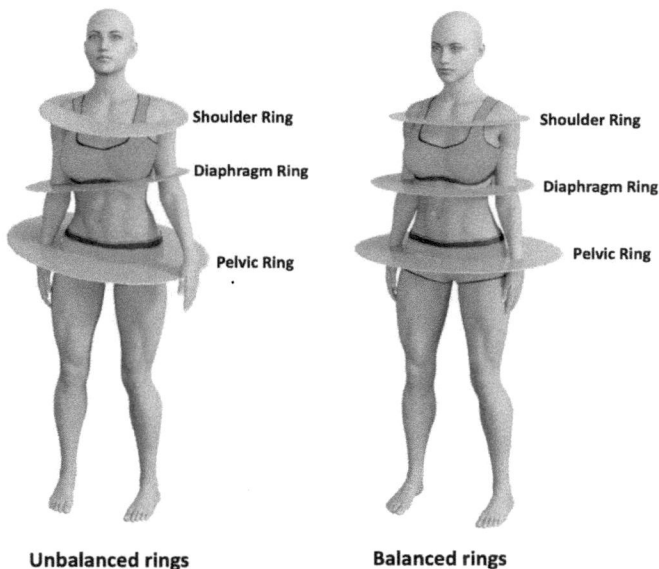

Shoulder Ring

Diaphragm Ring

Pelvic Ring

Shoulder Ring

Diaphragm Ring

Pelvic Ring

Unbalanced rings   Balanced rings

Figure 2: Three Rings of the Torso

It is particularly important that these three rings be balanced with each other, so the vertical polarity doesn't get stuck or diminished before reaching the head. If the rings are imbalanced, (e.g., not parallel while standing upright on both feet), then vertical polarity will not be allowed to move freely up. Pain and suffering are usually the result.

Most people live with contracted joints and aberrant or compensatory movement patterns, which greatly impairs their ability to move balanced and freely within gravity. Most people would agree that moving through water feels much freer than moving through air because the effect of gravity is diminished due to our bodies being less dense than water.

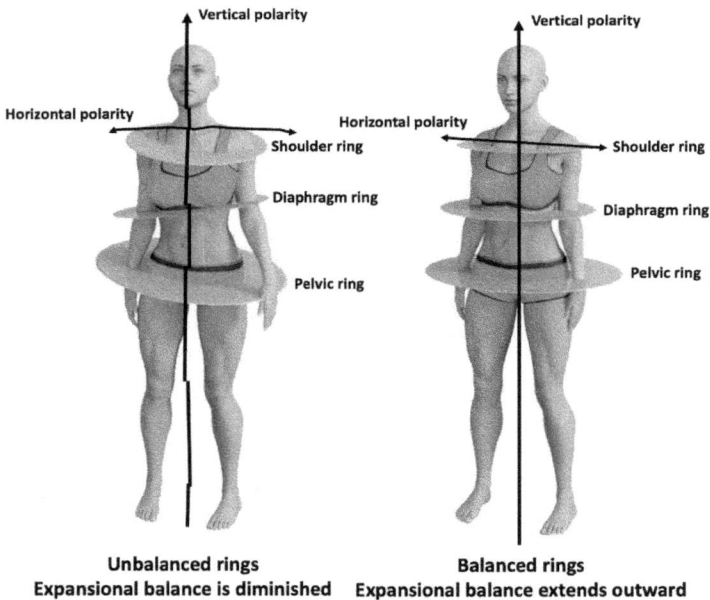

Figure 3: Expansional Balance

Expansional balance of the limbs is always counterbalanced by a place within the core from which the movement expands. This expansional balance is compromised when the body is not structurally integrated into a neutral position. Imagine water flowing through a tube. If that tube is twisted or kinked, then the water gets stuck and cannot flow freely. When the arms and legs are contracted or the torso and head are twisted from center, then the energy of expansion in response to gravity gets stuck, and the feeling of expansional balance is diminished. A lack of fluidity and movement is the result, which can lead to aches and pains and a lower quality of life.

Expansional Balance as a Concept

Let's recap the concept of expansional balance. Pelvic extension begins the vertical polarity and balances the pelvic ring. The pelvic ring then establishes a foundation for the diaphragm ring, balancing the lumbar area of the spine. The balanced diaphragm ring then establishes a foundation for the shoulder ring. The shoulder ring is a floating intermediary between the horizontal and vertical polarities that defines the sides of the body and allows the effortless extension of the head and neck. The head then naturally finds balance on the neck.

Expansional Balance:
A Fitness Regimen

The goal of this book is to illustrate basic exercises that combine strength, endurance, and flexibility into a health and fitness regimen that will generate a greater degree of expansional balance in the body. This is a far different perspective on health and fitness from training and conditioning the body to maximize performance. However, exercises carried out with expansional balance in mind will enhance order and function of the body, which will lead to greater performance.

Expansional balance is, in essence, about free movement of the joints. The exercises I've listed will help release tension and open the joints to allow freer, more fluid movement. An integrated feeling of the whole body can then be attained. Free movement in the joints is actually the function of our body's natural design. Poor patterns of movement, trauma, surgeries, disease, psychological conditioning, and other factors can cause us to lose that potential for ideal joint movement.

Any repeated movement will shape the body. Athletes, dancers, construction workers, and cubicle dwellers evolve their bodies according to habitual movement patterns. Some people become superbly efficient with their body mechanics. Some are slightly distorted, while other people's bodies are wrecked from their experiences. By combining strength, endurance, and flexibility into your workout regimen, you can structurally reorganize the body to address any distortions in your mechanics *and* maintain the new, improved organization.

The exercises in this book will release contracted fascia and bring awareness of aberrant holding patterns and compensatory movements. They will reorganize your body into a more efficient and neutral alignment. Reorganizing the body into a more efficient structure is not as much about building muscle but addressing the overall balance of the fascial webwork across the bones they stabilize. These exercises will ask you to look deeper to the bones and skeletal mechanics, rather than just build muscle like you would at the gym. Keeping the concepts of expansional balance in mind will also have you using the exercise machines at the gym in new ways—maybe different from how a fitness trainer would have you use them!

Last but not least, these exercises should be used as a guide rather than a recipe. You can apply the concept of expansional balance to any workout or exercise regimen.

CHAPTER 2

CORE AND SLEEVE

The exercises in this book are designed to improve the structural integration of the body's core and sleeve, which should be an essential aspect of any exercise regimen. What do I mean by "core" and "sleeve"? These terms may have different meanings depending on the context, and I define them in a way that's specific to structural integration.

The core is the deeper muscle and fascial layers of the body used to stabilize the torso so the limbs can move freely. The core is the area of postural movements that counterbalance the movements of the arms and the legs. The exercises in this book will expand, strengthen, and align the core with the rest of the body into a more efficient organization (i.e., neutral alignment).

The sleeve is the outer muscle and fascial layers of the body used for large and fast movements. The sleeve rides on top of the core (arms) or moves below the core (legs), while the core remains unobstructed by the movements of the sleeve. The exercises in this book will organize movement and restore strength and flexibility to these areas.

These exercises will rebalance many of the parts of the body (e.g., ankles, knees, hips, lower back, shoulders, and neck) that may be out of alignment. They will open the sleeve, organize the core, and integrate them. Said another way, *they will structurally integrate differentiated segments of the body so they can move as parts of a greater whole.*

CHAPTER 3

SELF-AWARENESS AND WILL

I n my experience as a massage therapist, the two main traits a person needs to create a lasting change are self-awareness and willpower. You can't move forward with just one trait; you need both. If a person is aware that a part of their life is unhealthy, then it won't get better if they lack the will to change it. Likewise, I've met people who have the will to exercise routinely, but no self-awareness that they're hurting themselves—high-performance athletes do this all the time. The connection between self-awareness and will is that they must be applied together.

The Power of Self-Awareness

The body is aware. It can listen and feel itself in space. Our bodies are designed with a network of nerve receptors for pressure, body position, and movement. But many of us have a reduced sense of self-awareness from years of moving or exercising in habitual ways.

Parts of the body that have been overcontracted for a long time may become withdrawn from our awareness.

The exercises in this book are designed with self-awareness in mind. With these routines, you will be moving the body in a manner that you wouldn't normally do on a day-to-day basis, which may even return some of the pleasant sensations you haven't experienced in movement for many years. Greater self-awareness will allow you to understand your habits and tendencies more clearly, both constructive and destructive. It will help you understand where you are weak, where you hold tension, and where you are unbalanced in your body. It will also guide you in how to work on those areas to improve your strength, endurance, flexibility, and ultimately quality of life.

By moving with greater awareness, you'll be able to harness the body's inherent plasticity—its ability to change. As you move through the rest of this book, I'll provide more guidance on how to carry out these exercises in a way that builds this crucial capacity for self-awareness.

What about Willpower? Sticking with an Exercise Routine

The benefits of having a regular exercise routine that will help you develop better self-awareness are huge: strength, endurance, flexibility, mood improvements, and on and on. What about the downsides of not having a routine? You might find yourself becoming weaker and slower, with less energy and a lower quality of life.

So how do you stick with this (or any other) routine? That's where willpower comes in. Willpower is important if you want to stick with any routine. But there's a lot of confusion out there about how to develop and maintain the willpower to do the things you know you need to do but may not always want to do. Thankfully, there's a key to developing your willpower. It's all about understanding how habits are formed and using that knowledge to your advantage.

Build Your Workout Willpower by Making It a Habit

So how do we develop the will to make exercise a daily part of our life? The answer is not motivational pep talks, discipline, goal setting, or making it fun. Even if we make exercise fun, eventually, like all regimental routines, it will cease to be fun—usually in a short period of time. The answer is *habit*! We're all creatures of habit. We create habits for getting ready for work, driving places, shopping, eating, and sleeping. Most of our lives are driven by daily patterns of repetitive routines. We turn those repetitive daily routines into habits for a reason: *to reduce our dependence on motivational processes*! That way, we continue to perform the repetitive routine even when it's not fun or pleasurable.

Yet the one thing that matters most in our lives, maintaining good health, is not part of most people's daily routines. The key to making exercise a part of your daily routine is to make it the highest priority. Your health must be thought of as the most essential thing in your life. Once you do that, then the decision to exercise or not becomes nonnegotiable. You'll just do it.

1. Write down your plan

First, you need the will to develop a regimented workout plan—I have provided several example plans later in the book. Find a workout plan and schedule that works for you and write it down. Verbally stating that you're going to set aside an hour each day for five days a week is fine, but you'll be more inclined to keep your commitments if you have them written down. Choose the right time in your schedule too. Try not to squeeze in a workout, not knowing if some other activity may interrupt your schedule. Plan ahead, and don't negotiate the time you have chosen.

2. Turn the plan into a routine

Once you have a plan written down, you can turn that plan into a daily routine. Start off slowly and understand your strengths and weaknesses. Don't take on too much at once. If you're just starting off, then maybe you don't want to join up with triathletes. Also, tell others what you're doing. If need be, have a talk with your spouse and other supportive members of your inner circle to give you the time and space to create a workout that fits your schedule.

Also, be kind to yourself and get plenty of rest. Physical and mental fatigue reduces your willpower to exercise. Getting enough sleep will ensure you're keeping your energy levels up.

3. Keep it up until your routine becomes a habit

Repetition is key to habit forming. If I continually do something over and over, then it can become a habit. In a study published in the *European Journal of Social Psychology*, Phillippa Lally, a health psychology researcher at University College London, and her team researched the process of habit formation in everyday life. They found that performing the same activity over and over resulted in forming automatic (habitual) behaviors within an average of a little over two months.

This time frame may sound daunting, but it should be inspiring. Don't fret if you're trying something new for a few weeks and you haven't mastered it yet. Making mistakes here and there won't have any measurable impact on your long-term habits. Don't worry if you break from your routine by a day or two. The stress from worrying is probably worse than the actual lost time. Forming a new habit is a process that takes time. Have faith in yourself, because if you do, you can accomplish anything. Once you have this new habitual behavior built into your lifestyle, it will become difficult to stop wanting to exercise.

Both self-awareness and will are personal. No one else can apply them for you. You must commit to exercising regularly. And when you exercise, you must be aware of your body's physical capabilities and actively engage those capabilities for a successful workout program. Use what you've read and learned (such as the guidance in this book), but ultimately trust your own needs, sensations, and experiences. The most successful workout program is one that is truly personalized.

Now that we've laid the important groundwork, let's move on to some warm-up exercises that will get your body ready for a vigorous workout.

CHAPTER 4

WARM-UPS

The following warm-up routine is a great way to start your workout session. It'll help open the rib cage to better fill the lungs with air during higher-intensity workouts, loosen your joints to prevent injury, and increase your circulation to bathe the muscle tissue with oxygen and nutrients during heavy lifting and/or exertion.

Deep Breathing

Intent: Expand your rib cage and increase your lung volume.

Start by standing with your feet parallel, about hip or shoulder width apart, whichever is wider. Find the pelvic extension (as described in the previous chapter) to extend the vertical polarity and balance the three rings of the torso. Center your body on the floor with your weight balanced through the centers of your feet. Use your awareness to judge if your weight is shifted either to the front or back of your feet and center it accordingly.

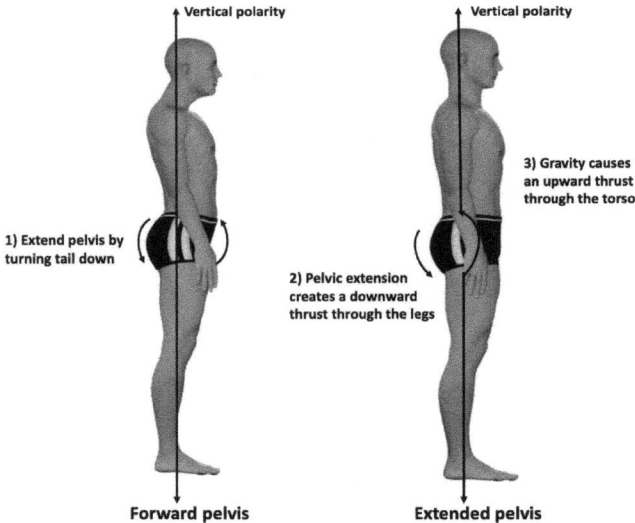

Figure 4: Vertical Polarity

When you find the pelvic extension, allow the crown of your head to rise as you begin to extend the vertical polarity. Imagine a string attached to the crown of your head that's being pulled up. This will relax the shoulders and allow them to fall back as well as allow your rib cage to expand. Relax your perineum (the region between the thighs below the pelvic ring, which surprisingly clenches up more than we realize!).

Now extend your arms out wide and to the side in a sweeping motion to open the rib cage, then raise them above your head while taking a deep breath. Place your palms face up over your head with your fingers overlapping. Hold your breath while spreading your elbows out. Imagine someone grabbing both elbows and pulling them behind you. Feel your chest expanding. Hold your breath for as long as it is comfortable (no turning blue in the face). Then, exhale slowly while lowering the arms to your sides. Continue to feel the string on the crown of your head being pulled up while you lower the arms. Repeat three to five times.[4]

Feel free to explore different ranges of motions with this warm-up. For example, while holding your breath and with elbows pulled back, rotate your body from the waist to the right and continue to hold. Then rotate back to center and exhale while lowering your arms back to your sides. Again, inhale while raising your arms, swinging them out to the side, and connecting your fingers above your head. Face your palms up while holding your breath, with your elbows pulled back, then rotate from the waist to the left side of your body and continue to hold your breath. Rotate back to center and exhale while lowering your arms back to your sides.

Another motion to explore: With hands overhead, palms up, and elbows pulled back, lean back and feel the stretch across the entire front of your body. Hold for as long as comfortable, then move back to center. Exhale and lower your arms to the sides.

---

4 I've written the number of repetitions or time spent holding a stretch, similar to following a recipe. However, feel free to do more or less, allowing your internal sensations to guide you.

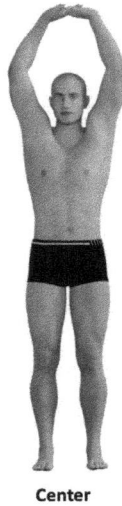

Center

Figure 5: Deep Breathing – Arms Overhead

After completing these motions, do a side bend while holding a deep breath with your hands over your head, fingers together and palms up. Return to center and slowly exhale while lowering your arms back to your sides. Repeat for the opposite side.

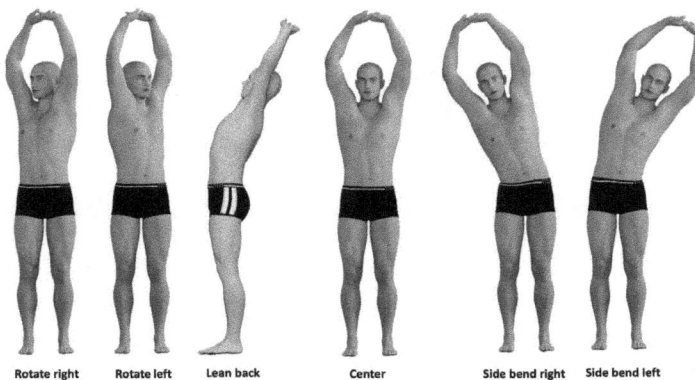

Rotate right   Rotate left   Lean back   Center   Side bend right   Side bend left

Figure 6: Deep Breathing – Rotate and Side Bend

Twisting at Waist

Intent: Open space in the spinal column for better circulation.

Now spread your feet a little farther apart, with both arms relaxed at your sides. Steadily (not forcefully), twist your upper body from left to right and back again. Continue in a rhythmic motion. Allow your relaxed arms to float freely across your midsection. Feel your spine twist with each turn from left to right. This motion will get the cerebral spinal fluid circulating.[5] Moreover, this motion will sometimes crack your back, release a lot of pent-up blockages, and increase space between the vertebrae. Continue for 10 to 15 seconds.

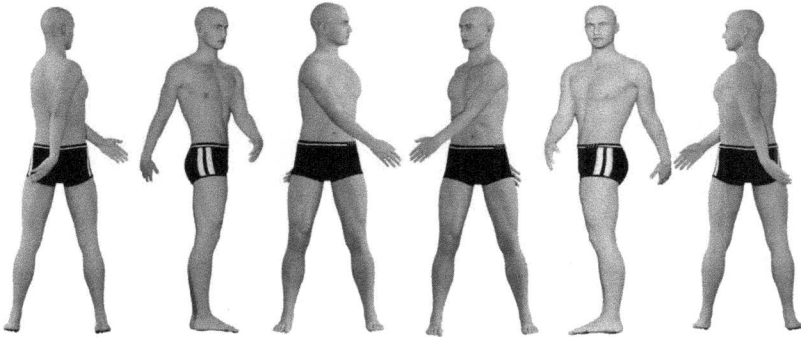

Figure 7: Twisting at Waist

5 Cerebral spinal fluid is a colorless fluid that goes around your brain and spinal cord, cushioning those organs, picking up nutrients from your blood, and removing waste products from brain cells.

Arm Swings

Intent: Loosen the shoulders and help free the head and neck from being pulled off center.

Continue standing in place, with feet parallel. Keep your hips in place and swing your arms in a crisscross motion from each other, swinging in front of and behind your body. While your arms are crossing in front of the body, alternate which arm lands on top of the other—right arm on top, then left on top, and so on. Continue for 10 to 15 seconds.

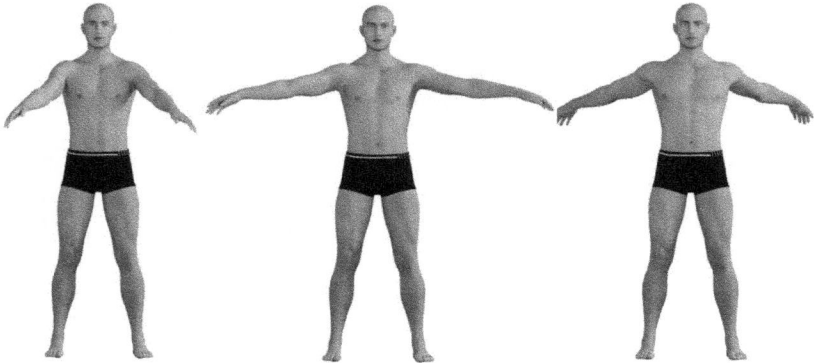

Figure 8: Arm Swings

Arm Circles

Intent: Extend the elbows from the spine, which frees up tension in the shoulder girdle and balances the shoulder ring.

Spread your feet a little farther apart, with both arms out to your sides. Remember, the extension of the arms from your torso comes from the elbows (like that of the knees extending from the pelvis). The arms are segmented, and I want you to feel that segmentation with this movement. Try to feel your elbows extending out from your spine through your shoulders, forearms from your elbows, and your wrists from your forearms. Imagine the shoulder girdle is a free and balanced yoke above the ribs. Check your awareness: In raising the arms, are you keeping the shoulders and neck muscles independent, or are you engaging the neck muscles to raise your arms? The latter can indicate chronic tension or aberrant holding patterns, which will create an imbalance with the shoulder ring. Imagine there is a core feeling of expansion coming from the chest, through the center of each joint, and out through the hands.

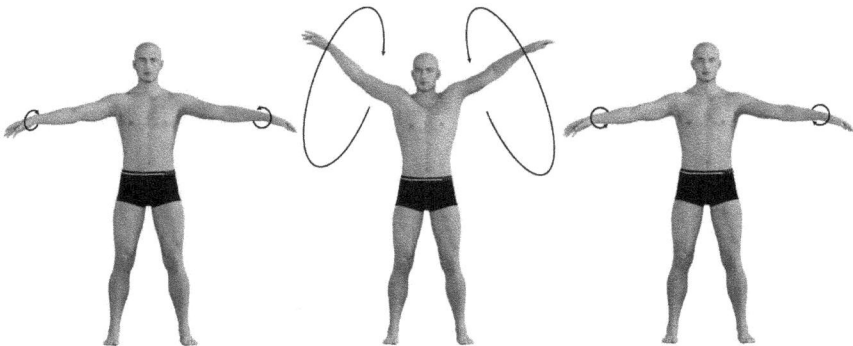

Figure 9: Arm Circles

Begin moving each arm in tiny circles. Gradually make the circles larger until each arm is fully swinging in its shoulder joint's mechanical limit. Then reverse direction. Gradually make the circles smaller and smaller until you're back to moving your arms in tiny circles.

This movement will free up tension in the shoulder girdle and increase circulation from the chest through the shoulders and into the hands. Repeat the warm-up by moving your arms in the opposite direction.

Shoulder Circles

Intent: Loosen the cartilage surrounding the shoulder joint.

Let's not stop loosening those shoulders. After all, your shoulders are working for almost all upper body exercises. Again, standing with feet parallel and arms to the side, find the pelvic extension and start rotating your shoulders in a circular motion. After three to five rotations, begin a circular motion with the shoulders in the opposite direction. Continue to rotate your shoulders in both directions for 20 to 30 seconds.

Only the shoulder girdle should be making this movement; the arms should be limp. Check your awareness: Are your arms stiff or even trying to aid in this movement? If so, this could be another sign of chronic tension that is creating imbalances in the shoulder ring. You should be able to feel the gristle grinding in your shoulder girdle, especially for older adults. Continue to rotate, changing from clockwise to counterclockwise as much as is comfortable.

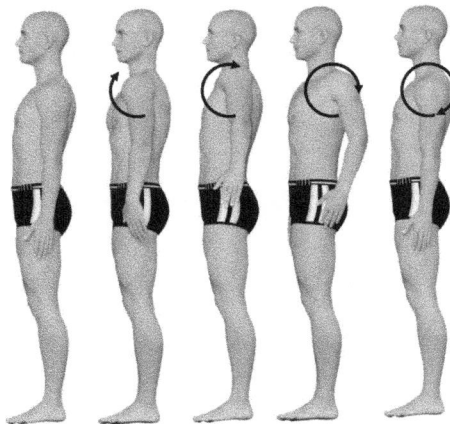

Figure 10: Shoulder Circles

Backward Palm Lock

Intent: Loosen the external fascial layer around the rib cage and release tension in the shoulder girdle, allowing the ribs to expand more freely with each breath.

Standing with feet parallel, find the pelvic extension, then interlace your fingers behind your back and push the palms of your hands together. Then stretch your arms out and lock your elbows. Hold this pattern for as long as it is comfortable (30 to 60 seconds). This motion will open your chest and whole shoulder girdle. It might be difficult, especially if you haven't been stretching for a while. Don't worry if you can't do it and allow yourself to make adjustments. For example, try not pushing the palms of your hands together, not locking your elbows, or both.

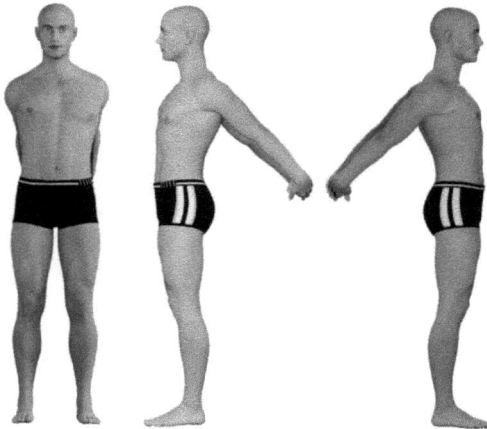

Figure 11: Backward Palm Lock

Head and Neck Roll

Intent: Free the neck from the shoulder girdle and differentiate the head from the neck.

I prefer to do this motion while locking the palms of my hands behind my back, but that isn't necessary. You can do this motion with your arms to your side as well. Imagine a pencil sticking straight out from the crown of your head. Draw a circle in the air above your head using the imaginary pencil. Then draw a circle in the opposite direction. Take care to not roll your head behind your back such that your eyes are looking up, as this just compresses the cervical spine. You're centering your head and neck over your shoulders with each circle. Continue this motion for 10 to 15 seconds. For older adults, you'll feel the gristle in your neck. This circular motion will loosen the cartilage around the cervical spine.

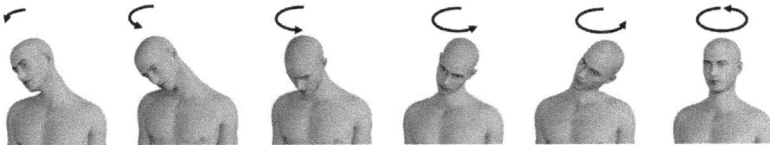

Figure 12: Head and Neck Roll

Next, bring your head back to center, with the crown of your head being pulled up by your imaginary string. Turn your head as far to the right as it can go and hold that position for five to ten seconds. Then rotate your head to the opposite side as far as it can go and hold again.

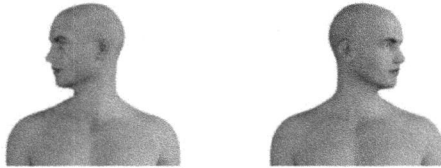

Figure 13: Head Turn

Check your awareness. Can you roll your head and neck independent of the shoulder girdle? Are you pulling the shoulder girdle with the rotation of your head? If so, then possibly the shoulder girdle is being drawn upward toward the neck by extrinsic muscles not necessary for this movement. The neck is often bound into the shoulder girdle, causing an imbalance with the weight of the head being off center of the body. Continue to practice these movements to differentiate the neck from the shoulder girdle and the head from the neck.

Full Pelvic Extension

Intent: Feel how the movement transmits your energy to extend down through the legs and into the feet, as well as upward through the spine and into the crown of the head.

This next warm-up is important because it balances the pelvis, which relates the hip joint to the lumbar spine. This movement improves the inherent structural integration of your whole body along the central axis of the core.

Standing with feet parallel about hip or shoulder width apart, keep your knees locked and take in a deep breath while bending forward at the hips and letting your hands fall as far down to (or onto) the floor as they will go. Relax your neck and shoulders and allow your head to drop.

Now slowly exhale and return to a standing position. The movement is first made by tucking your pelvis under and pushing your feet into the ground. You'll have to unlock your knees midway up to allow your pelvis to continue to turn down. Imagine the pelvis is a universal joint between the legs and the spine. The lift of the spine is created when the pelvis is turned down, which turns the downward push through the feet into the upward thrust of the spine.

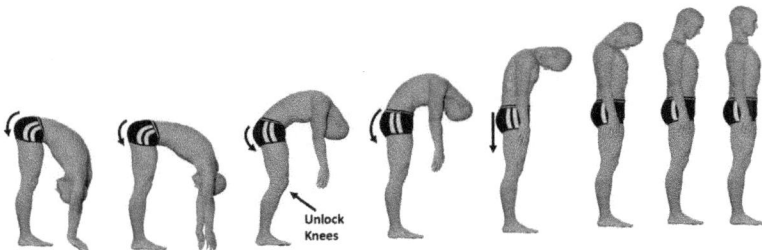

Figure 14: Full Pelvic Extension

As you rise back up, feel your vertebrae stacking on top of each other one piece at a time, with the head lastly stacking on top and finding its balance on top of the neck. Gain a sense of "arrived" when your head has turned up and the movement is completed. Do this motion three to five times or as many more as you like. This is a great movement to loosen your hips and lengthen your spine, allowing your pelvis to become better organized into a more neutral position.

Standing Hamstring Stretch

Intent: Release tension in the hamstrings to allow the pelvis to move more freely and balanced across the hip joint.

Spread your feet apart about hip or shoulder width, whichever is wider. Take a step forward with the right foot and turn the left foot slightly out. With one hand on the left knee and another on the lower right leg, bend the left knee while keeping your right leg straight and knee locked. Be sure to keep the right foot flat on the ground.[6] Bend far enough over to feel the stretch in your hamstrings.

Next, shift your weight to combine movement between the bent knee and your hips so you can pivot and rotate slightly at the right ankle joint (which is why you want to keep the right foot flat on the ground). Play with the movement of the hip and bent knee to gain awareness of where most of the tension in the hamstrings is located. Tension in the hamstrings can cause the pelvic ring to tilt forward. Once you get a sense of where that tension is located, hold the position and concentrate on stretching that area for 30 seconds.

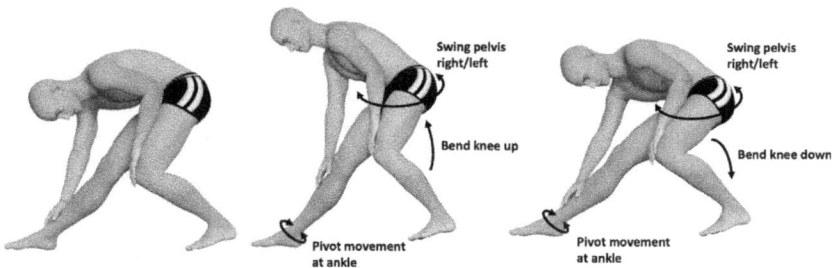

Figure 15: Standing Hamstring Stretch

6 In the classical way of teaching the standing hamstring stretch, the ankle is bent with the toes pointed up, which further stretches the hamstring attachments on the fibula. In this version of the stretch, we want to instead pivot the ankle and hip joints simultaneously to discover where tension is located in the hamstrings.

Transition to Inner Groin Stretch

Intent: Expand the knee from the groin area.

Continue to hold the standing hamstring stretch for the right leg (per the above description). Pivot your left foot to point your toes behind you and bend at the knee to lower your whole body closer to the floor. Next, place your elbow in the pocket of the inner knee and use the elbow to push your left knee as far away from yourself as you can to open up the groin area. This motion will lengthen the inner muscles of the thighs.

Keep your right foot flat on the ground if possible. It's okay if the heel comes up off the floor. As time goes on and you become more flexible, eventually you'll be able to do this stretch while keeping your foot flat on the floor. Hold the position for 30 seconds.

Repeat the standing hamstring stretch and transition to the inner groin stretch for the other leg.

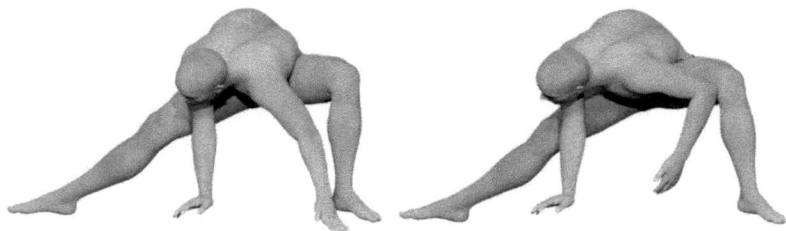

Figure 16: Inner Groin Stretch

Quad, Shoulder & Neck Motion Combo

Intent: Loosen the muscles in your upper leg and increase circulation in the shoulder and neck.

You can practice this warm-up standing with no assistance, but I prefer to have one hand against a wall or some other support. With your right hand supported, grab your left ankle with your left hand. The focus is on lengthening the quadriceps of the left leg. Imagine a string attached to the front of the kneecap (which is now pointed down), with something pulling that string straight to the floor. Don't bring your knee behind your back, as this will engage additional muscles that are not the focus of this warm-up.

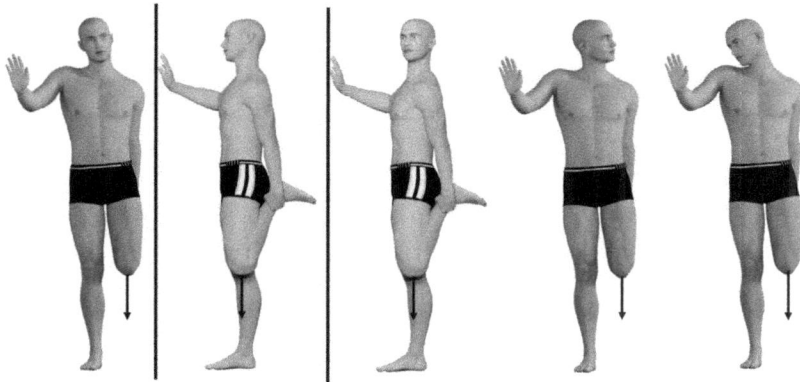

Figure 17: Quad, Shoulder & Neck Motion Combo

While the imaginary string is pulling your knee to the floor, feel your left shoulder being pulled along with it as you continue to hold the left ankle. This is a good time to slowly rotate and bend your head to the right. Feel the muscles in your neck getting taut and notice where the greatest tension is. Explore different movements with your neck (such as rotating or bending it) to work out any excess tension, either in your neck or shoulder. You should be able to feel your shoulder being pulled in two directions at once.

Continue this motion for 30 seconds, then repeat the steps for the opposite side.

Calf Stretch

Intent: Open the ankle joints, allowing your feet to become better grounded under the weight of the body.

With two hands against a wall, put both legs out behind you. Gently drop the left knee forward while bending at the right ankle. Stretch the lower right leg just enough to feel the calf muscles begin to tighten. Slowly and gently straighten the left knee and bend the right knee forward, this time bending the left ankle. Feel the stretch in the left calf muscle.

Rhythmically alternate between stretching the right and left calf muscles. Continue this back-and-forth motion for 15 to 30 seconds. Check your awareness. The calf muscle will start to lengthen, and the ankle will open. You'll be able to increase the bend at the ankle and/ or increase the tension in the lower leg as this happens. The motion should not be forceful or painful.

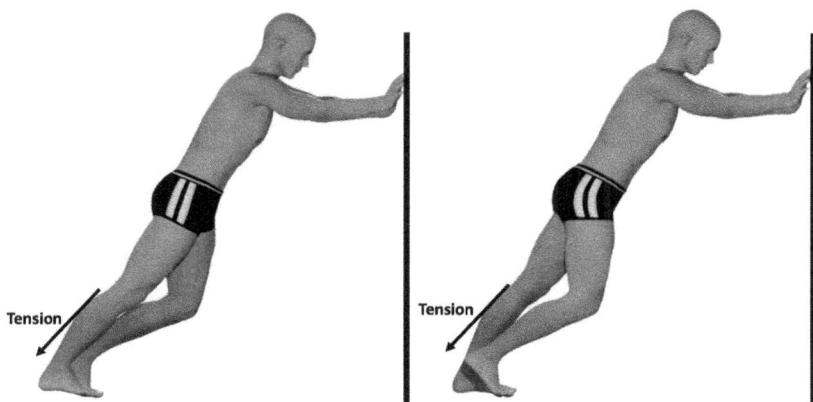

Figure 18: Calf Stretch

Ankle Rotations

Intent: Open the ankle joints and establish balanced movement of the foot on the ankle. Organizing the feet also releases length up the back.

Keep the same position as the calf stretch, but now you're going to put just your right toes on the floor. This works best with shoes on. Pivot your entire ankle in a circular motion. Start by slowly turning the ankle clockwise for three to five complete rotations. Then turn your ankle counterclockwise for three to five complete rotations. Continue to slowly rotate your ankles in both directions for 15 seconds. Like above, this motion should not be forced. Repeat for the left ankle.

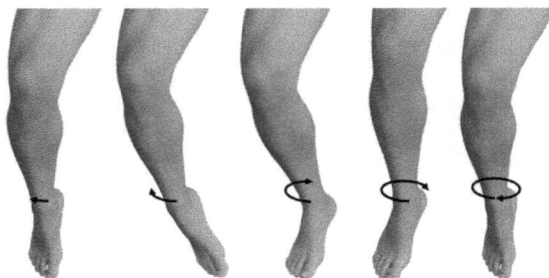

Figure 19: Ankle Rotation Clockwise

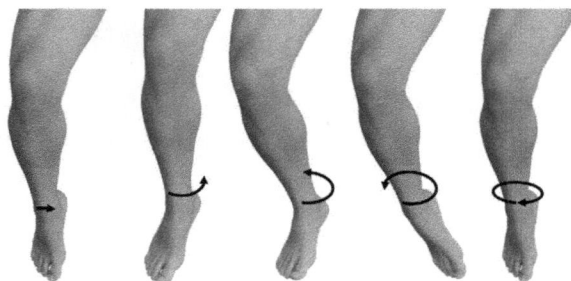

Figure 20: Ankle Rotation Counterclockwise

Now that your joints are properly lubricated and your body is warmed up, you'll be more enthusiastic to begin an intense workout. Moreover, this warm-up routine is not only a great way to start your workout session, but a great way to start your day. I invite you to do it every day for one week and see how much better you feel!

CHAPTER 5

STRENGTH

A strength building exercise is any physical activity designed to improve muscular strength and fitness by exercising a specific muscle or muscle group, either by lifting, pushing, or pulling against an external resistance. External resistance can include free weights, your own body weight, weight machines, resistance tubing, or resistance bands. Also, exercising for strength can be done at home or in the gym, with a friend or by yourself. There are so many choices to make when creating a fitness regimen to build and maintain muscular strength, and thankfully you can apply the ideas and methods in this book to any form of exercise you choose. That's what's great about this approach. It's up to you to determine which exercises and equipment are right to incorporate into your own fitness regimen.

This section of the book will focus on *engaging the muscles to create better skeletal alignment of the joints and building strength to stabilize the joints* (think bones). You are not trying to maximize muscular gain! Maximizing muscular gain is what a person normally understands and teaches for strength training. Instead, this book *emphasizes raising your awareness and fully integrating and balancing all the body's joints.*

Methods of Strength Building

There are so many ways to describe how to build and maintain strength. There's powerlifting larger weights with shorter repetitions to gain muscle mass. There's using less weight with more repetitions to gain muscle growth and endurance. Then there's the question of frequency: how many circuits to do as well as how many days a week to perform the exercise? It's up to you to answer these questions and develop your own personalized exercise regimen. Moreover, this doesn't mean you have to rely on one method exclusively. Alternating different methods may be the best approach for long-term success, as it allows you to get the benefits of a range of strength building exercises.

Of course, you should use self-awareness to understand what approach your body responds to best. The strengthening exercises I describe here are only a few examples of over a thousand different ways to build strength. I've chosen these exercise examples because combined, they constitute a full-body workout that engages all the skeletal muscles and joints of the body. You may eventually wish to create your own exercise regimen for building and maintaining strength using the method and equipment you're most comfortable with, armed with the knowledge of expansional balance. Therefore, instead of telling you to use a particular resistance machine, I'll list the muscle or muscle group that engages during that specific movement. Using the concepts of expansional balance, you can come up with an exercise method that mimics that movement using the external resistance of your choice.

Building Awareness of Habitual Patterns of Muscular Tone Development

When a motion of the body is executed, it is not an isolated event. Many of the muscles in the surrounding areas, if not the entire body, also must be initiated to support the motion. When the body is at rest, the muscles ideally have a minimal level of tone. But when, for example, you raise a leg to walk, many muscles must contract and others lengthen, while they *all* maintain a steady level of tone so that the motion does not cause a dislocation at the joint. Additionally, many muscles must increase their tone to create the bracing necessary to keep your body from falling over due to the overbalanced side. When the leg is raised, the muscles of the whole body must adjust their tone settings to maintain the new posture. Now if the leg is to continue moving forward, a whole new set of muscle commands imposes another layer of stimulus pattern, which must compensate to the conditions of a fixed shoulder girdle, imbalanced torso, outstretched arm, and forward-tilting neck and head.

At birth, we are all born with an initial level of muscular tone, which maintains the integrity of our bodies. As we grow, our tone levels increase to accommodate the increase in tension from moving longer, heavier limbs. As we mature even more, we develop our own ways of doing things to maintain our posture and gait. As we repeat these habitual patterns of movement in an effort to stay upright, they become our "norm." But this new norm often creates distortions and imbalances in the "tone settings" that shape the patterns of muscular tension throughout the body (e.g., tighten the neck forward here, relax there to drop the chest, alter here to turn a knee out to the side, or tilt the pelvis a little due to a slumped back). These imbalanced muscular tone settings shape our bodies, and our tensions become as unique to each of us as our fingerprints. Moreover, as we grow older our habitual muscular tone can become more and more unbalanced.

Ultimately, we want to move away from unhealthy habitual patterns of movement. *In order to restore healthy and balanced muscular tone, we need to exercise our muscles in a way that we wouldn't normally do in our daily activities.* General strength and muscular tone can be gained by varying the use of our muscles. Be cautious of systems of exercise being taught that frame a repetitive process as being perfect or best (including this book). A solid workout program should contain enough variation to build and maintain greater strength and balance of muscular tone.

What is needed to accomplish this goal is awareness: awareness of our habitual patterns of movement, awareness of areas of our body that are conditioning those patterns, and of what it would feel like if our patterns of movement were different. With this awareness, you can begin to correct, strengthen, and expand the joints out from your core and through the sleeve to create greater expansional balance.

Building Strength for Coordinated Movement and Balance

When we think of strength building exercises, we think of muscle. Lifting weights or doing resistance exercises will help to gain strength, which means bigger muscles. We often think of muscle strength and contraction as the sole functions of the muscle. However, controlled muscle *lengthening* is key to coordinated movement and balance. Therefore, the focus of these strength building exercises is for you to move segmented body parts together smoothly and efficiently (coordination), as well as to keep control of your body without falling over (balance).

Building Strength to Stabilize Joints

The skeleton is held erect by muscle. Muscle supports the joints. Stability of the joints is maintained above all by the activity of the surrounding muscles. Ligaments also play a part, but they will stretch and loosen under constant strain when muscles are weak. Therefore, building and maintaining strong muscles can help improve posture, function, vitality, and normal activity.

Strengthening Goals

One of the goals of all these strength exercises is to complete a full range of motion (ROM) during the exercise. The difference between training for maximum strength gain and the concepts taught in this book is that we want to concentrate on *bones*, not muscles. This may sound contradictory, but it's not. These exercises will still strengthen the muscles, but they will also stabilize the joints and organize the bones to be in a more neutral and integrated alignment with the entire skeleton. Exercising through the full range of motion of the joints will aid in both stabilizing the joints and organizing the bones into this improved alignment.

Upper Body: Core and Sleeve

The intent of upper body exercises is to connect the upper limbs (sleeve) to the spine (core) through the shoulder girdle. The arms are also the counterweight to the upper pole of the head. Every movement of the arms has a reference within the core. Therefore, we are trying to establish a balance across the entire shoulder ring.

Chest Press and/or Incline Press

Intent: Balance the shoulder girdle while pushing the arms forward of your chest.

Concentrate on a smooth and balanced motion of the shoulder girdle sliding across the chest, extending through the arms and hands above the chest. Does the shoulder girdle have an open balance, or is there tightness, causing restricted breathing? Concentrate on integrating the arms during the whole movement. Can you feel if the arms are rotated from your wrists and hands? Are the elbows or a locked shoulder causing a twist in your outward motion? Is one side (or one joint) not quite the same as the other? For example, is the left arm stronger than the right, causing the barbell to slope down to the right side of your body? With this awareness, you can begin to correct and strengthen the right arm by balancing the movement through the whole shoulder girdle. Complete 10 to 12 repetitions per set for three sets each with approximately 30 seconds between each set. Complete a full range of motion, focusing your attention on the targeted muscles.

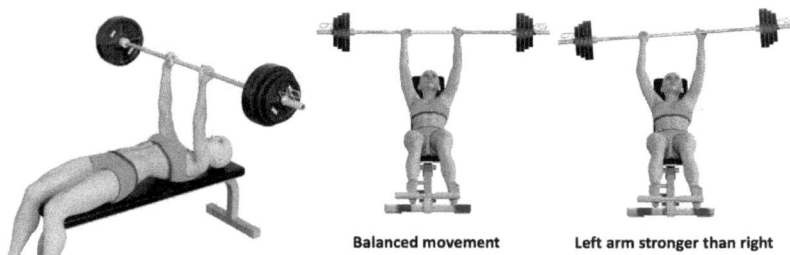

Balanced movement   Left arm stronger than right

Figure 21: Chest Press and/or Incline Press

Muscles targeted: anterior deltoids, middle deltoids
(incline press), pectoralis major, triceps

Overhead Press

Intent: Balance the shoulder girdle while pushing the arms above your chest.

The overhead press is similar to the chest press, only now we're engaging a few different groups of muscles. Concentrate on the shoulder girdle moving freely in a smooth and balanced manner on the sides of the chest with arms extending above the head. Feel the movement coming from inside the shoulder joint. Are your shoulders raised toward your ears? This could be a sign of chronic tension in your upper shoulders that's restricting your shoulder joints from opening. With this awareness, you can begin to correct, strengthen, and expand out from your core by balancing out the movement through the whole shoulder girdle. Complete 10 to 12 repetitions per set for three sets each with approximately 30 seconds between each set. Complete a full range of motion, focusing your attention on the targeted muscles.

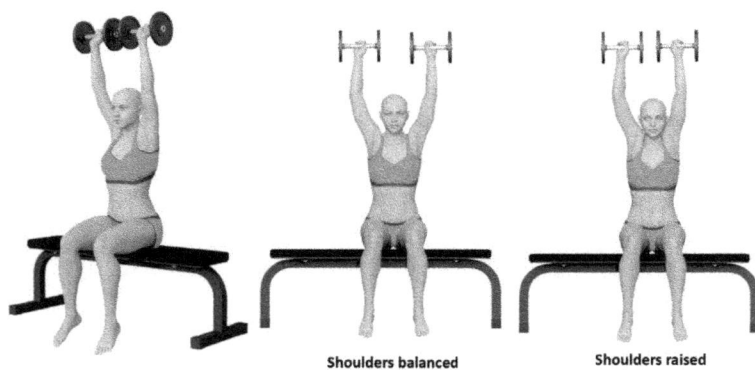

Shoulders balanced   Shoulders raised

Figure 22: Overhead Press

Muscles targeted: middle deltoids, upper trapezius, middle pectoralis, triceps

Pull-Back

Intent: Balance the shoulder girdle while pulling the arms behind your chest.

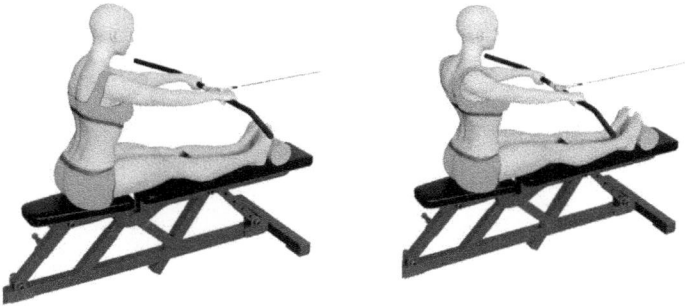

Figure 23: Pull-Back

Muscles targeted: rhomboids, posterior trapezius, middle pectoralis, triceps

Concentrate on a smooth and balanced motion of the shoulder girdle. Pull-backs can have a variable connection to the spine. Remember that the core counterbalances the sleeve. Depending on whether you're moving with your elbows and wrists slightly above or below your shoulders, the stabilization may come from any part of the back. When the elbow is above the shoulders, the arm is balanced from the lower area of the spine. When the elbow is below the shoulders, the arm is balanced from a higher area of the spine. While performing this exercise, alternate your elbows to be above and below your shoulders and concentrate on the area of your spine that is pulling and stabilizing the shoulder girdle. Bring your awareness to your spine. Are you pulling with your arms instead of your back? If so, then you're not allowing the shoulder girdle to move freely behind your chest. Complete 10 to 12 repetitions per set for three sets each with approximately 30 seconds between each set. Complete a full range of motion, focusing your attention on the targeted muscles.

Lateral Raise

Intent: Isolate the joints of the shoulders so the elbows can move up or down and extend out freely from the core.

Concentrate on a smooth and balanced upward and downward motion of the elbows extending through the shoulder girdle. While performing this exercise, do you sense if your elbows are moving freely up and down beginning at the shoulder joint, or is the movement coming from your neck and upper shoulders? If so, that could be a sign of chronic tension in your neck and upper shoulders, which will constrict free movement of the head. Complete 10 to 12 repetitions per set for three sets each, with approximately 30 seconds between each set. Complete a full range of motion, focusing your attention on the targeted muscles.

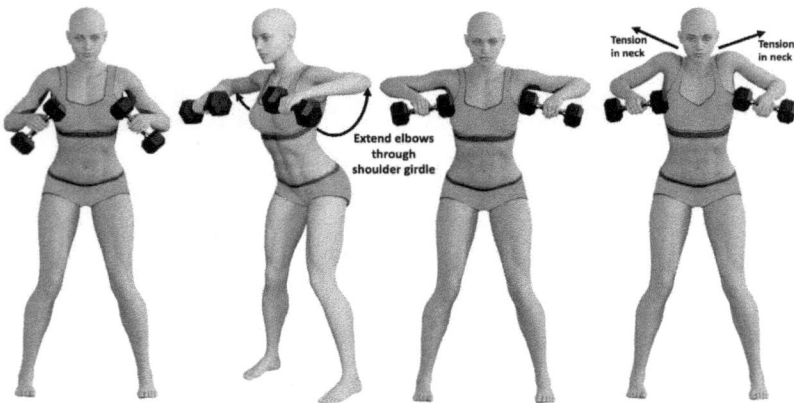

Figure 24: Lateral Raise

Muscles targeted: upper trapezius, middle deltoids, levator scapula, supraspinatus/infraspinatus, serratus anterior

Pull-Down/Chin-Up

Intent: Stabilize and balance the shoulder girdle sliding across the top of your core with the arms pulling down below your chin.

Concentrate on a smooth and balanced motion of pulling the arms down from above your head. During this exercise, find the interior connection coming from deep down the sides of your torso and from your lower back. Can you feel where, if any, expansional balance is not happening? Feel if there is tightness in the shoulder girdle (e.g., scapula does not rotate freely) or somewhere deeper in the core (e.g., relying on strength of the biceps rather than engaging the lower trapezius to complete the exercise). Complete 10 to 12 repetitions per set for three sets each with approximately 30 seconds between each set. Complete a full range of motion, focusing your attention on the targeted muscles.

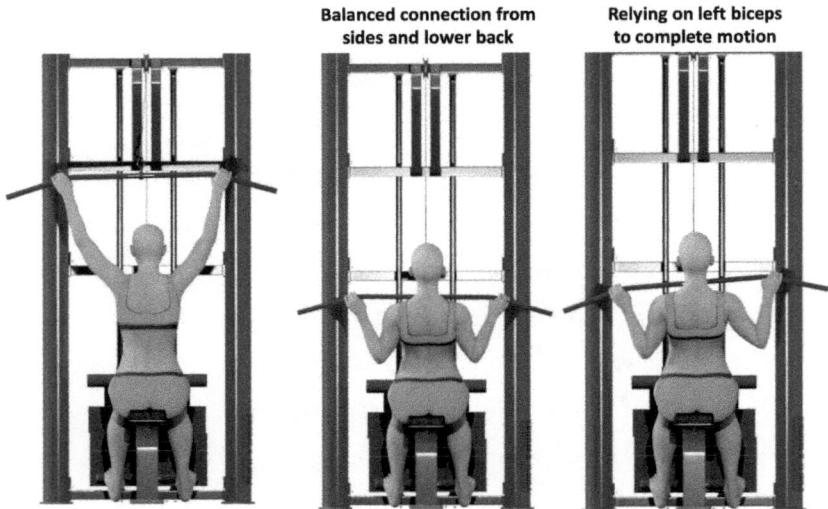

Figure 25: Pull-Down/Chin-Up

*Muscles targeted: latissimus dorsi, lower trapezius, biceps brachii,
brachialis, pectoralis minor, teres major, rhomboids*

Pectoral Fly

Intent: Organize the upper and lower balance of the shoulder girdle while moving your arms across the front of your body.

Concentrate on a smooth and balanced motion of bringing the arms front and center of your chest. Bring your attention to the shoulder girdle sliding across the chest with your arms extending out from the spine through your elbows and into your hands. Does it feel as though the muscles in your arms (sleeve) are trying to complete the movement? The tension should be coming from the torso (core). The movement should be extending out from the front of your core at differentiating points of counterbalance between the torso and upper sleeve. Complete 10 to 12 repetitions per set for three sets each, with approximately 30 seconds between each set. Complete a full range of motion, focusing your attention on the targeted muscles.

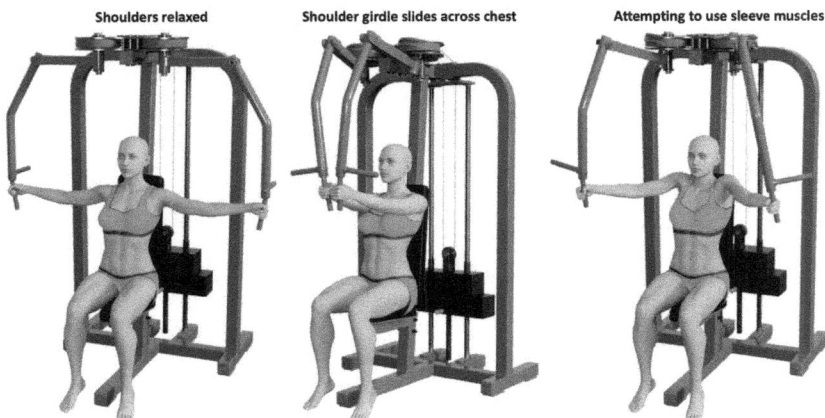

Figure 26: Pectoral Fly

Muscles targeted: pectoralis major, anterior deltoids, coracobrachialis, biceps (short head)

Rear Deltoid Fly

Intent: Similar to the pectoral fly, organize the upper and lower balance of the shoulder girdle, except now the movement is extending out from the back of your core along the spine.

Concentrate on a smooth and controlled motion of pushing the arms back, starting from the front of your body and out to your sides. Notice if your shoulders are rising toward your ears. This could be a sign that your shoulder girdle is not balanced and you are attempting to use other muscles to compensate. Complete 10 to 12 repetitions per set for three sets each, with approximately 30 seconds between each set. Complete a full range of motion, focusing your attention on the targeted muscles.

Balanced shoulders   **Shoulders rising**

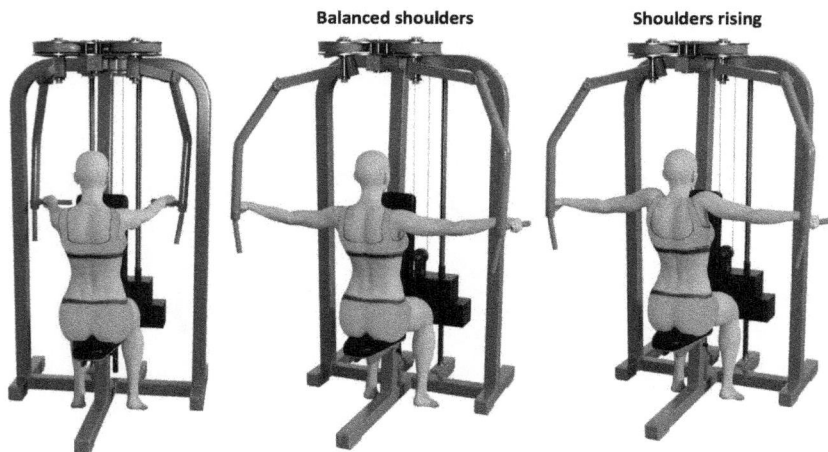

Figure 27: Rear Deltoid Fly

Muscles targeted: supraspinatus (initiates movement),
lateral middle deltoid, posterior deltoid

Dip

Intent: Stabilize the joints of the whole shoulder girdle.

This exercise engages the entire shoulder girdle. One advantage of this exercise is that it will engage opposing muscle groups at the same time while developing overall upper-body strength. Notice if one shoulder leans farther forward or backward than the other. This could be a sign that one side is weaker than the other and thus out of balance. You should feel a stretch in your chest as you're doing this exercise. Complete 10 to 12 repetitions per set for three sets each, with approximately 30 seconds between each set. Complete a full range of motion, focusing your attention on the targeted muscles.

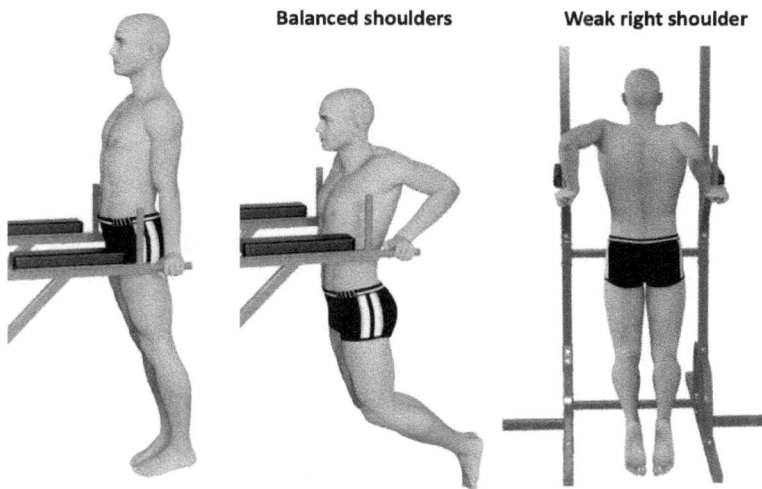

Balanced shoulders   **Weak right shoulder**

Figure 28: Dip

Muscles targeted: triceps, anterior/middle deltoids, pectoralis major/minor, latissimus dorsi

Abdominal: Core

The focus of these core exercises is to establish a front-to-back balance across the torso as well as lengthen the spine. Think of the core as a series of segmented hinges that fold out to an extended form. The core begins with the inner thighs connecting to the pelvis, which when balanced correctly, releases the pelvis to find a new flexible connection with the lumbar spine and extends upward through the shoulder girdle and up the head and out the arms.

Stomach Crunch

Intent: Strengthen the abdominal muscles, balance the pelvis and lumbar spine, and hold the abdominal contents in place while making breathing easier.

The front portion of the abdominal wall is the rectus abdominis. The proper function of the rectus abdominis is to lift the pelvis and assist the diaphragm and lumbar spine from the front during any position of spinal flexion or extension. Proper functioning of the rectus muscle (while the pelvis is horizontally aligned) is necessary for the vertical expansion of the lumbar spine.

Moreover, the rectus abdominis also has a unique relationship with breathing, evidenced in its fascial connections with the diaphragm and its role as a regulator of hydrostatic pressure in the abdominal cavity. The rectus can control breathing by forcing exhalation when the muscle is tightened and causing inhalation when it is released.

From the point of view of expansional balance, the exercise is done by lifting the rectus at various points, differentiating its segments. Complete a single set of 50 to 75 repetitions, focusing your attention on the targeted muscles.

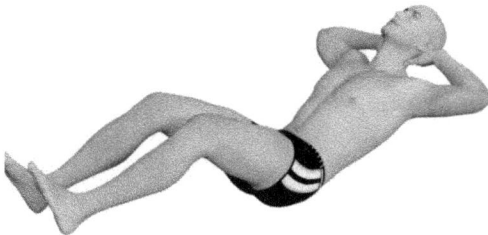

Figure 29: Stomach Crunch

Muscles targeted: rectus abdominis

Rotating Sit-Up

Intent: Build rotational strength and pelvic stabilization.

Similar to the sit-up, this is a basic core exercise with an added rotation. It can be done on the floor or on a machine or bench, with or without the feet anchored. Take care not to hyperrotate as this can cause undue pressure on the vertebral disks. I prefer to keep one leg crossed over the other and bring my knee up and cross the opposite elbow. This ensures that I'm not hyperflexing while twisting the spine. Notice if your breathing is difficult, which could be a sign of weak respiratory muscles. Complete a single set of 20 to 35 repetitions, focusing your attention on the targeted muscles.

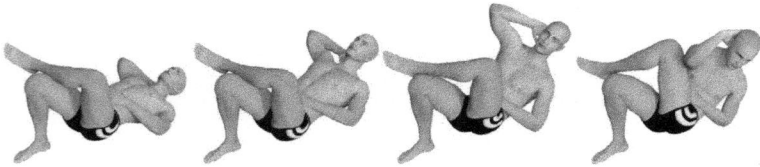

Figure 30: Rotating Sit-Up

Muscles targeted: external obliques

Leg Lift

Intent: Create a balanced flexion and extension between the rectus and the psoas

Leg lifts are great for building and maintaining core strength and balance, which leads to better body control. The psoas often becomes chronically shortened, pulling the lumbar spine forward and compromising the balance of the entire torso. This exercise helps to strengthen and differentiate the lumbar hinges in relation to the pelvic extension. Notice if there is any pain in the lower back. This could imply weakness and/or tightness of the lumbar hinge. I prefer to place my hands directly under my sacrum to ensure an extension of the pelvis during this exercise. Complete a single set of 20 to 50 repetitions, focusing your attention on the targeted muscles.

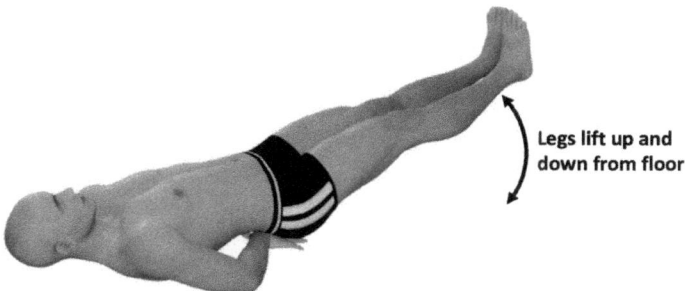

Legs lift up and down from floor

Figure 31: Leg Lift

Muscles targeted: rectus abdominis, psoas, quadriceps

Side Bend

Intent: Establish a sense of the sides of your body. Clarify which muscles are in the front of the body and which ones are in the back.

The oblique muscles of the abdominal wall participate in lifting or lowering different segments of the rectus muscle. You'll need to concentrate on keeping the pelvis still while raising your torso. Feel the tension on the sides of your body.

Notice if your body is attempting to twist or the pelvis is rising. This could be a sign of weak muscles in the sides of the lower back. It's important to note that side bends only work in a tiny range of motion. Complete 10 to 12 repetitions per set for three sets each, with approximately 30 seconds between each set. Complete a full range of motion, focusing your attention on the targeted muscles.

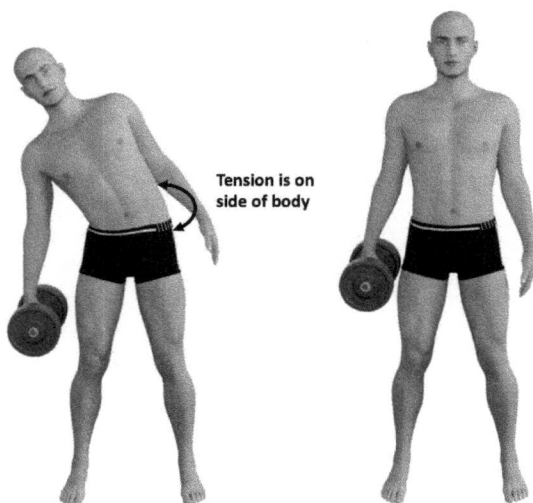

Tension is on side of body

Figure 32: Side Bend

Muscles targeted: external/internal obliques, quadratus lumborum, erector spinae

Back Extension

Intent: Balance the sacroiliac joint so that the pelvis is stable and does not tilt off center.

Back extensions are important for building and maintaining lumbar strength, which supports and balances the lumbar sacroiliac joint. Again, think bones, not muscles. There are so many ways to complete this exercise (e.g., lifting just the upper back, lifting the legs and upper back simultaneously while lying on the ground, using machines or a bench, etc.). As stated above, it's up to you to develop some familiarity with this exercise and perform it the way you're most comfortable.

Notice if there is trembling or wiggling in your body when performing back extensions. This could be a sign of weakness that's causing an imbalance with the pelvis. Work on strengthening the lumbar sacroiliac joint to improve the function and balance of the pelvis. Complete 10 to 12 repetitions per set for three sets each, with approximately 30 seconds between each set. Complete a full range of motion, focusing your attention on the targeted muscles.

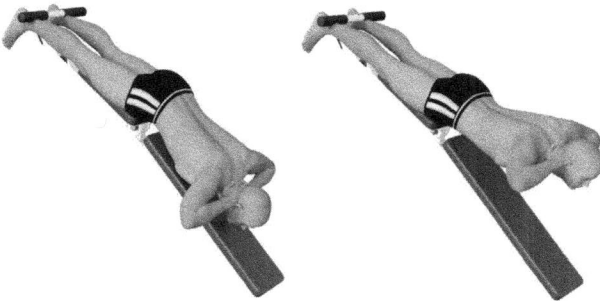

Figure 33: Back Extension

Muscles targeted: erector spinae

Arms: Sleeve

The arms are designed to extend out from the shoulder girdle and be the counterweights to the head and neck. If an arm is shortened or twisted at its segments, then the entire limb is affected all the way up to the shoulder girdle. The free extension of your arms is essential to the upward extension of the head and neck. Remember, the body is not simply a fluid wave of expansion. The expansion occurs across segments.

The focus of these exercises is twofold. First, they will give the arms a sense of a horizontal expansional balance extending from the core through the segments of the shoulder, elbow, and wrist, which will create smooth, effortless overall movement. Second, they will build strength in each segment of the arms, which will aid in balancing the horizontal polarity freely along the side planes of the body.

Biceps Curl

Intent: Build and maintain strength of the biceps and maintain a strong counterbalance for the head and neck.

There are so many ways to complete a biceps curl (e.g., free weights, machines, tension bands, sitting or standing, etc.). I'm just going to give one example; however, you'll want to use the concept of expansional balance with whatever method you choose. In this example, using free weights and a curl bar, stand with feet parallel about hip or shoulder width and find the vertical polarity in your body as described previously. Maintain the vertical polarity while focusing on engaging just the targeted muscles.

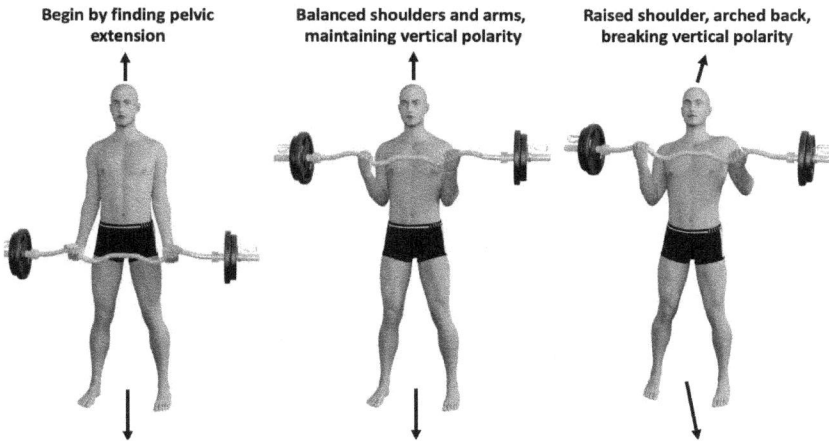

Begin by finding pelvic extension   **Balanced shoulders and arms, maintaining vertical polarity**   **Raised shoulder, arched back, breaking vertical polarity**

Figure 34: Biceps Curl

Muscles targeted: biceps brachii, brachialis, brachial radialus

Focus your awareness on isolating the targeted muscles while flexing the forearm up. Notice if your body is trying to use the shoulders or moving your torso forward and/or backward (rocking motion) to aid in the lifting. If so, then this could be a sign of chronic tension that's causing your arms to be drawn up toward your head and neck, contracting the horizontal polarity rather than extending it. Complete 10 to 12 repetitions per set for three sets each, with approximately 30 seconds between each set. Complete a full range of motion, focusing your attention on the targeted muscles.

Triceps Curl

Intent: Build and maintain strength of the triceps and maintain a strong counterbalance for the head and neck.

In this exercise, raise and lower a dumbbell behind your head to exercise the triceps, either sitting or standing. Complete a full range of motion while maintaining the vertical polarity. The biceps and triceps act against one another to bend and straighten the elbow joint. You want to focus your awareness on isolating the targeted muscles while extending the forearm up. Bring your attention to the shoulder girdle, with your arms extending out from the spine through your elbows and into your hands. Notice if one arm is weaker than the other. This can result in unbalanced movement at the segments of the arms, negatively altering the horizontal polarity. Complete 10 to 12 repetitions per set for three sets each, with approximately 30 seconds between each set. Complete a full range of motion, focusing your attention on the targeted muscles.

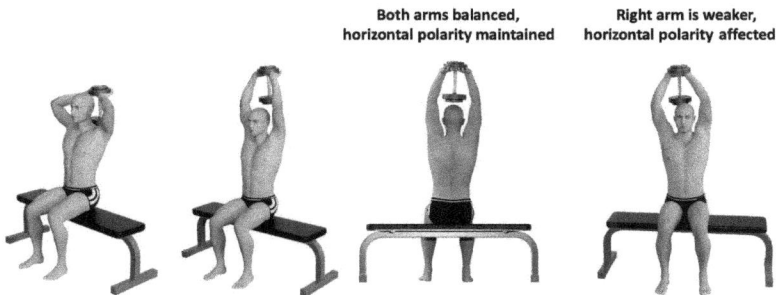

Both arms balanced, horizontal polarity maintained

Right arm is weaker, horizontal polarity affected

Figure 35: Triceps Curl

Muscles targeted: triceps

Forearm Curl

Intent: Build and maintain strength of the segments of the forearms and wrists.

Like the biceps curl, there are many ways to complete a forearm curl. I'm only going to describe one method, but you can use the concepts of expansional balance with whatever method you choose.

Using free weights and a curl bar, perform curls to exercise the flexor muscles and then the extensor muscles of the forearm. To allow for expansional balance, the hands must extend out from the shoulder girdle and through the elbow to make contact with the environment. Notice if you're attempting to draw your arms up into your shoulder girdle while performing these exercises. Again, this can be a sign of chronic tension that's limiting horizontal extension through each of the segments of the arms. Complete 10 to 12 repetitions per set for three sets each, with approximately 30 seconds between each set. Complete a full range of motion, focusing your attention on the targeted muscles.

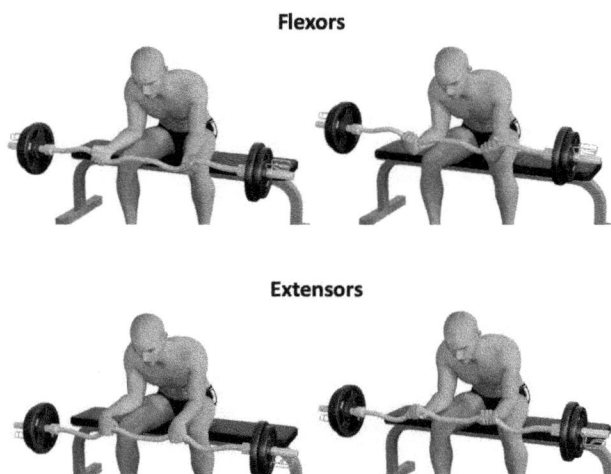

Flexors

Extensors

Figure 36: Forearm Curl

Muscles targeted: anterior (flexor) and posterior (extensor) compartments of the forearms.

Legs: Sleeve

The core rides on top of the legs and depends on the legs to stabilize the pelvis and maintain balance. Moreover, the legs extend from the core in a segmented design. The expansion of this segmented design is critical to stabilize the pelvis and balance the core. If any of the segments of the legs are withdrawn or twisted, the integrity and balance of the core will be compromised.

The expansion of this segmented design is clearly displayed when taking a step. The knee initially expands out from the spine and through the pelvis. The second expansion comes from the hip out to the ankle, counterbalancing across the knee. The expansion continues from the knee to the inside arch of the foot, then from the tarsal arch to the toes. If any part of the leg is shortened or twisted at its segments, then the entire limb is negatively affected all the way up to the core.

These exercises have two goals. First, to work the leg muscles to create a more balanced alignment of the joints at each segment. Second, to build and maintain strength in the legs, which will aid in the vertical expansion of the body and stabilize the pelvis.

Leg Extension

Intent: Strengthen and organize the front of the knee joint to balance the alignment of the legs between the hips and the ankles.

While performing leg extensions, make smooth, isolated movements (without engaging your upper body). Bring your awareness to the tension moving through the center of the knees while keeping your toes straight up and not twisted out to the side. Is there any pain? Are your feet twisted out to the sides? This could be a sign of hips chronically turned out, affecting the balance of the pelvis. If so, then use less resistance to keep your legs more aligned while performing this exercise. Complete 10 to 12 repetitions per set for three sets each, with approximately 30 seconds between each set. Complete a full range of motion, focusing your attention on the targeted muscles.

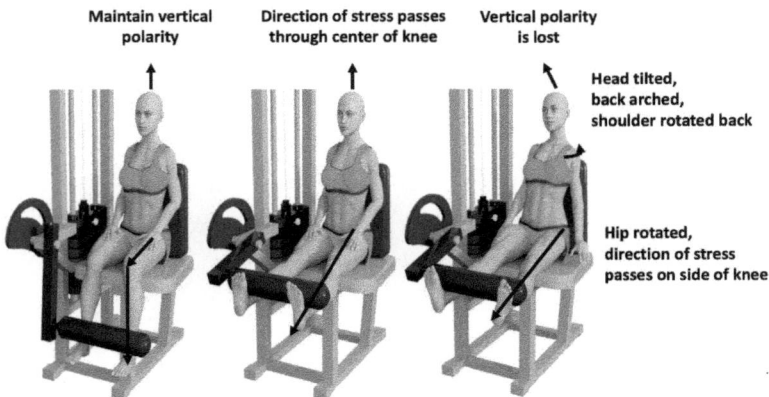

Figure 37: Leg Extension

Muscles targeted: quadriceps

Leg Curl

Intent: Strengthen and organize the back of the knee joint to balance the alignment of the legs between the hips and the ankles.

While performing leg curls, focus your awareness on the backs of your upper legs. Is one side weaker than the other? Is your pelvis twisting off center during the exercise? This could be a sign the muscles are weak and not properly stabilizing the pelvis. If so, then use less resistance to keep your legs more aligned while performing this exercise. Complete 10 to 12 repetitions per set for three sets each, with approximately 30 seconds between each set. Complete a full range of motion, focusing your attention on the targeted muscles.

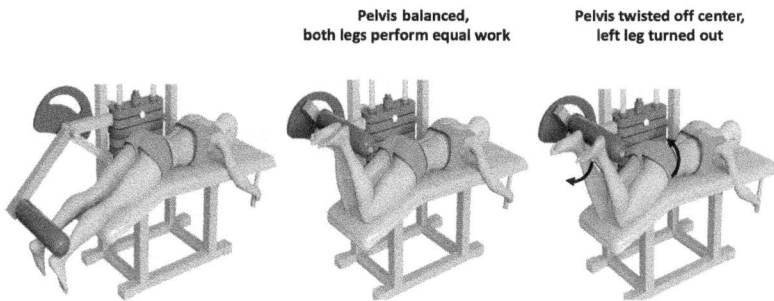

Pelvis balanced, both legs perform equal work

Pelvis twisted off center, left leg turned out

Figure 38: Leg Curl

Muscles targeted: hamstrings, popliteus

Leg Press (Squat)

Intent: Establish a ground connection that begins at the heel and travels up the legs through the pelvis and into the spine.

This is an exercise that is usually taught in a manner to increase the size of your muscles by turning your feet out, which can train the muscle to support hyperturnout of the hips. This method is fine if your intent is to maximize muscular gain. However, we are instead working on engaging the muscles to create better alignment of the joints as well as build strength to stabilize the joints (think bones). Keep your focus on the fullest possible connection between the pelvic extension and the lumbar balance while performing this exercise.

When squatting down, allow the backs of the legs to let your knees float forward, keeping your knees over your toes and your feet parallel. When standing up, you're not so much pushing the weight up, but instead feel your feet dropping into the ground. The downward thrust of the feet into the ground creates the upward thrust of the spine.

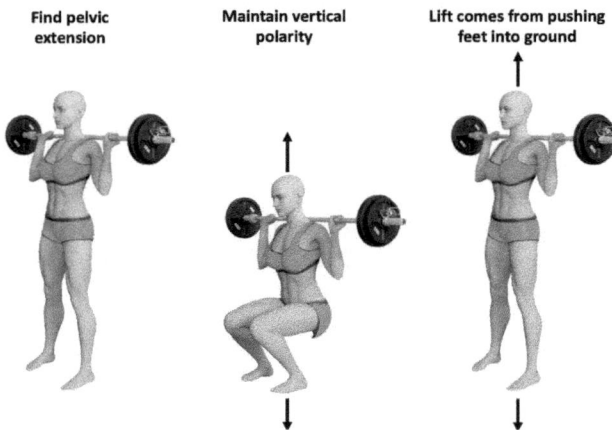

Find pelvic extension   **Maintain vertical polarity**   **Lift comes from pushing feet into ground**

Figure 39: Leg Press

Notice if you are balanced or feeling wobbly while performing this exercise. Can the legs move while the pelvis remains stable? This could be a sign that your legs muscles need to be strengthened. Are there rotations in the knees or ankles, causing imbalance? Are you shifting your weight over to one leg? Being aware of these things will allow you to avoid the risks and damage associated with these patterns of movement. Complete 10 to 12 repetitions per set for three sets each with approximately 30 seconds between each set. Complete a full range of motion, focusing your attention on the targeted muscles.

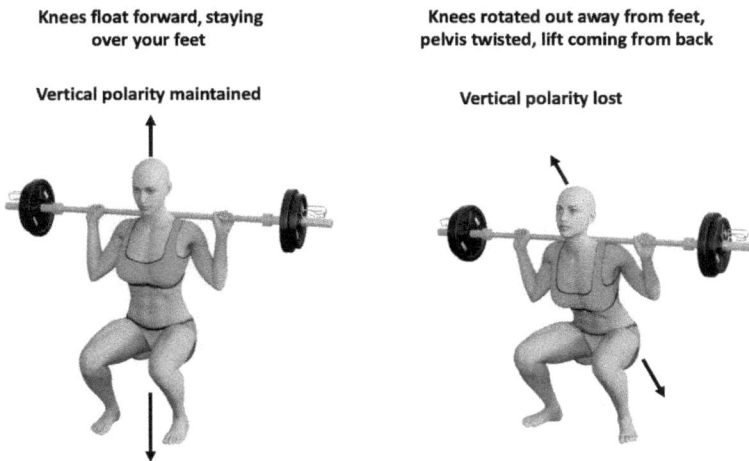

Knees float forward, staying over your feet

Knees rotated out away from feet, pelvis twisted, lift coming from back

Vertical polarity maintained

Vertical polarity lost

Figure 40: Leg Press – Vertical Polarity

Muscles targeted: gluteus, hamstrings, quadriceps

Calf Extension

Intent: Build and maintain strength of the segments of the lower leg and stabilize the ankles.

All the weight of the body is supported by the calf muscles and tendon straps that wrap under the feet to create the arches of the feet. Weak ankles can affect your balance, which can lead to chronic instability. Notice if your ankles are twisted or rotated while performing this exercise (e.g., shifting your weight on the outside of your foot or the ankle can cause your foot to turn inward). This could be a sign of weak, unbalanced ankles. Complete 10 to 12 repetitions per set for three sets each, with approximately 30 seconds between each set. Complete a full range of motion, focusing your attention on the targeted muscles.

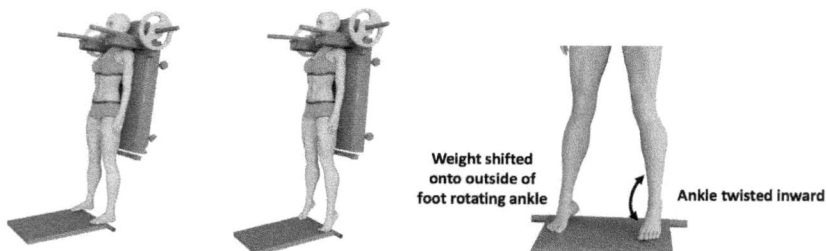

Weight shifted onto outside of foot rotating ankle

Ankle twisted inward

Figure 41: Calf Extension

Muscles targeted: soleus, gastrocnemius

Hip Adduction

Intent: Stabilize the hip joint.

Hip adductors help stabilize the pelvis and balance the knees. They are the reciprocal hip muscles to the abductors. When walking, bring your awareness to your hips. Notice if your hips are turning out while walking, which could be a sign of hip adductor muscle weakness. Complete 10 to 12 repetitions per set for three sets each, with approximately 30 seconds between each set. Complete a full range of motion, focusing your attention on the targeted muscles.

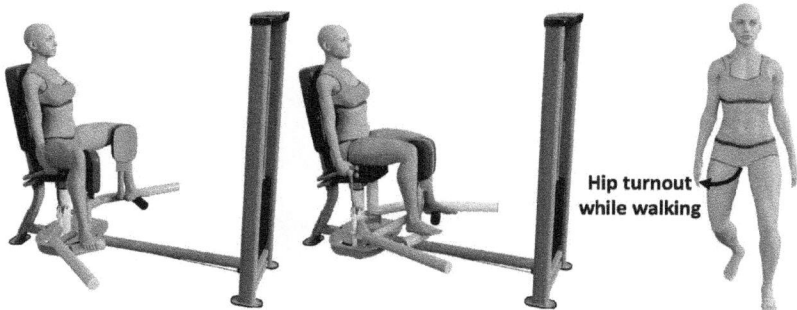

Hip turnout while walking

Figure 42: Hip Adduction

Muscles targeted: adductor longus, gracilis, adductor brevis, adductor magnus, pectineus

Hip Abduction

Intent: Stabilize the hip joint.

Every time we take a step with one leg, the opposite hip joint must abduct to keep us upright. When walking, bring your awareness to your hips. Does one hip drop down? This could mean weakness in the opposite hip abductors. Or do you waddle when you walk? This may indicate weakness on both sides. Complete 10 to 12 repetitions per set for three sets each, with approximately 30 seconds between each set. Complete a full range of motion, focusing your attention on the targeted muscles.

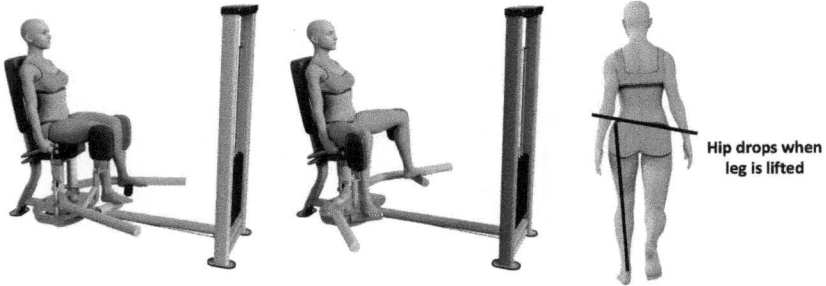

Hip drops when
leg is lifted

Figure 43: Hip Abduction

*Muscles targeted: gluteus medius, gluteus minimus,
tensor fasciae latae, piriformis, sartorius*

Great job getting through the strength portion of your exercise regimen. Your muscles are pumped, your bones are stronger, and your joints are more open and stable. Now it's time to get your sweat on with some high-energy endurance exercise.

CHAPTER 6

ENDURANCE

Now that you're done with the strengthening portion, it's time to move on to aerobic (or endurance) workouts. Aerobic exercises are full-body activities of varying intensity that increase the heart rate. The benefits are numerous, from an increased sense of well-being and less emotional stress, improved circulatory and respiratory systems to weight loss.

The concepts of expansional balance can be applied to aerobic exercises just as well as the strength and flexibility exercises. While doing these exercises, keep your focus on finding the pelvic extension to begin the vertical polarity. Then relate that extension to the lumbar balance. Then find the horizontal polarity by opening the shoulders and arms. The head will naturally find balance on the neck. If you keep these steps in mind, then your aerobic exercises will result in expansional balance, enhancing the structural order and function of your body. Any exercise without it will just cause the three rings of the torso to become unbalanced. Aches, pains, and stiffness in the joints will be the result.

There are a slew of aerobic workouts that build and maintain endurance, such as burpees, jumping rope, jumping jacks, squat jumps, kickboxing, dancing, running, and brisk walking, just to name a few. In this book I'll cover just three examples: brisk walking, running, and cycling. Whatever workout you choose, I recommend that you maintain an increased heart rate that causes you to break out into a sweat, for 30 minutes per day and a minimum of five days a week. This will help to ensure a healthy level of endurance.

Brisk Walking

Intent: Aid in releasing tension and opening up the joints to allow freer, more fluid movement within them.

Brisk walking is a low-intensity exercise that can help you maintain a decent level of aerobic endurance depending on your level of fitness. Focus your awareness on tracking the gait of your body. When walking, point with your knees in the direction you intend to go. The feet should be tracking parallel with each other, not turned out to the side or inward. This will aid in maintaining a stable pelvis, which will translate into extending the vertical polarity. Also, the core should stabilize the torso, counterbalancing the movement of the arms and legs. The legs should be moving freely within the hip joint, not swinging out to the side. The arms should be riding on top of the core, so the core remains unobstructed by their movements.

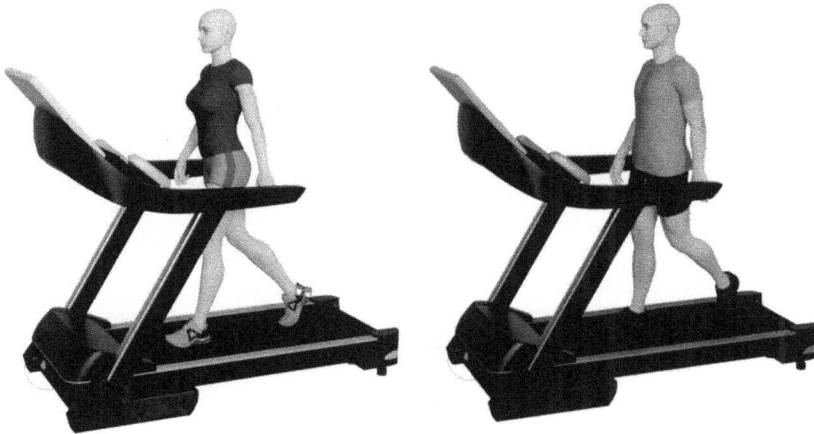

Figure 44: Brisk Walking

Jogging/Running/Sprinting

Intent: Build and maintain an efficient level of function to move longer, harder, and faster.

Jogging, running, or sprinting will increase the level of aerobic intensity (sprinting being a very high level of intensity). The tone of the muscles will increase to ensure the bracing of your joints and to keep your body from falling over. While jogging, running, or sprinting, notice if the shoulder girdle is opened, allowing the horizontal polarity to extend into the elbows. Is your head tilted to the side or balanced on top? Use your awareness to correct aberrant patterns of movement and attempt to adjust accordingly.

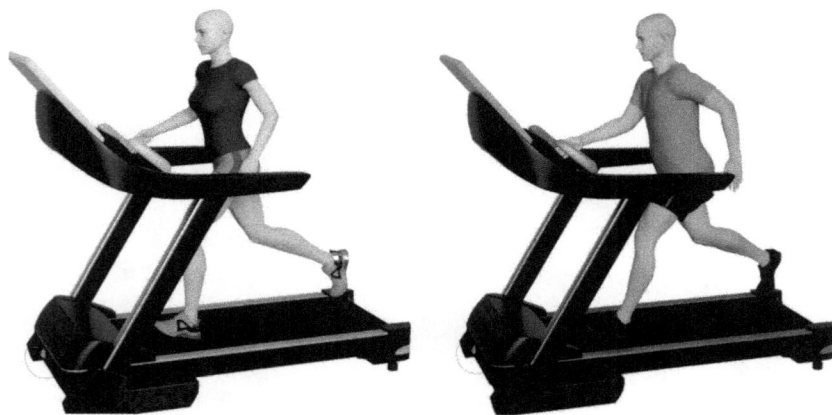

Figure 45: Jogging/Running

Bicycling/Stationary Bike

Intent: Aid in releasing tension and opening up the joints to allow freer, more fluid movement within them. Build and maintain an efficient level of function to move longer, harder, and faster.

Cycling is a great aerobic exercise that doesn't put much impact on the skeletal joints, as opposed to running. Moreover, cycling is a great alternative for those who may have conditions that prohibit them from engaging in a high-impact exercise regimen.

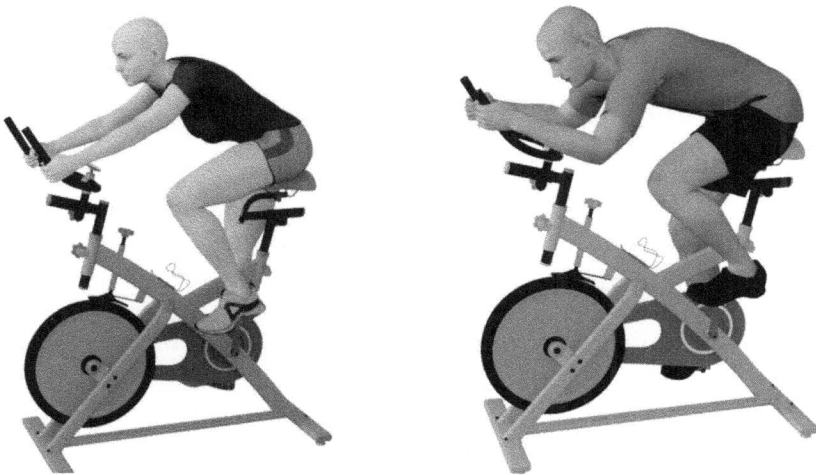

Figure 46: Bicycling/Stationary Bike

Many trainers and coaches will give advice on improving performance for cycling, such as clipping the balls of your feet to the pedals, then tucking your body in and holding your spine in place to transfer the energy down to your legs to make them spin faster. (Imagine a figure skater holding her arms out while spinning. As she draws her arms in, she then spins faster and faster.)

This is great advice if you wish to compete with others. However, that advice is counter to opening the joints and allowing freer, more fluid movement. When cycling with expansional balance in mind, as in standing, the vector of force pushing down with your leg comes from the pelvis and through the arch of your foot, not the ball of your foot. The point is not to force the energy of momentum down into the legs, causing them to spin faster. The energy of momentum needs to expand naturally outward through the spine, shoulders, and head.

Let's look at how cycling with expansional balance works in a little more detail. The pelvic extension causes a downward force. The reaction force (resistance from the bicycle) exerts an upward force that lifts the spine. Since the downward force is coming from only one leg (instead of two as in standing), it will cause the upward force to exert a bend to the spine on the opposite side of the leg that's pushing down. In turn, the bent spine will cause one shoulder to rise. This back-and-forth undulating movement (as you're pedaling) loosens the hips, the pelvis, and the spinal column and opens the shoulder girdle, thus achieving greater structural organization with the three rings of the torso.

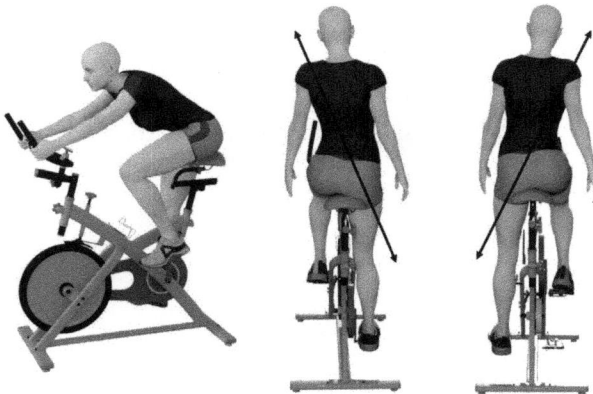

Figure 47: Stationary Bike – Maintain Pelvic Extension

A high-intensity cardio workout can temporarily boost your flexibility because it increases circulation to your muscles and joints. But it also puts strain on those muscles and joints, which can lead to stiffness later, so let's move on to the flexibility exercises to help keep you moving easily and comfortably.

CHAPTER 7

FLEXIBILITY

Building and maintaining flexibility is critical to any health and fitness program. I've been doing these exercises since I was nine years old. I've also been working out at health and fitness clubs (still doing these exercises) since I was 18. What astonishes me the most in this industry is the lack of attention to stretching by physical fitness coordinators, personal trainers, and gym enthusiasts. Many gyms and health and fitness clubs don't even create a space for their members to stretch. Most fitness books I've read will maybe bury a small comment in the text on the benefits of stretching. However, the importance of stretching cannot be overstated. Stretching is just as important as strength building and cardiovascular exercises and should be given equal time (if not more time for older adults) out on the gym floor to create and maintain a healthy body.

Connective Tissue/Fascia Continuity

The goal of this book is to establish a new perspective (expansional balance) that can provide a clearer understanding of the structure and organization of our body. One aspect of that clearer understanding would be the relationship of the connective tissue with the muscles and bones. A brief description of connective tissue is therefore needed.

"There is no tissue in the body that is as ubiquitous as connective tissue, and as it migrates and develops in various forms in various locations, its 'connective' qualities cannot be overstated. Connective tissue binds specific cells into tissues, tissues into organs, organs into systems, cements muscles to bones, ties bones into joints, wraps every nerve and every vessel, laces all internal structures firmly into place, and envelops the body as a whole. In all of these linings, wrappings, cables, and moorings it is a continuous substance, and every single part of the body is connected to every other part by virtue of its network; every part of us is in its embrace." (Deane Juhan, *Job's Body* 1987, pp. 62–63)

From this perspective, connective tissue can be seen as the *prima materia* of the body. It's the most basic and holistic system in the body, both connecting and separating all other elements. This continuity would imply that there are no truly local effects or events in the body.

As people get older, connective tissue (e.g., myofascial tissue, ligaments, and tendons) stiffens and even shrinks (called creeping) with age. The amount of collagen and elastin in connective tissue decreases, usually due to a loss of tissue water content or systemic disease. These tissues become drier, less elastic, and more prone to injury or "snapping." As a result, joint motion decreases and the risk of injury increases. Older men are especially prone to these connective tissue changes, which is why more men than women generally complain about decreased flexibility and joint pain.

Chronic tension and scarring (due to injury, trauma, or surgery) will also reduce the flexibility of the connective tissue. Like a sweater that is pulled in one direction, the connective tissue adjacent to the point of the pull will stretch out in the same direction. These factors can affect muscular alignment and cause aberrant patterns of movement.

The good news is that a large part of the loss of flexibility and increase of stiffness is due to lack of use. Remember the old saying, "If you don't use it, you'll lose it." Well, if you haven't been, then start using it! Stretching can reverse much of the tightness and aches associated with aging. If you're already stretching, then congratulations and keep doing it!

Myofascial tissue stretches are held continuously for at least 90 to 120 seconds. This is how long it takes for the fascia to begin to let go. Shorter stretches do not affect the collagenous aspect of the fascia (connective tissue) and therefore lead to only temporary, partial results.

Muscular Stretch Reflex

When a muscle lengthens, the muscle spindle is stretched and its nerve activity increases. This increases alpha motor neuron activity, causing the muscle fibers to contract and thus resist the stretching. This stretch reflex, or more accurately "muscle stretch reflex," is a contraction that functions to maintain the muscle at a constant length. A secondary set of neurons causes the opposing muscle to relax. Holding the stretch anywhere from ten seconds to three minutes allows enough time to "reset" the stretch reflex and elongate connective tissue.

Stretching with Awareness

Personal awareness is important while stretching. If you go into a stretch and you're not feeling a release, then you may need to spend more time easing into it. Give your body time to relax into the position. Breath comfortably, and your nervous system will realize what's happening and allow the tissue to elongate. This is especially true if you're working a specific area to ease tightness, heal an injury, or achieve a goal, such as the splits.

Coming out of a stretch should not be painful. However, with more intense stretches, you will need to come back to neutral position slowly. The main takeaway is to feel and understand your limits so you know when you've done enough.

Stretch Routine Examples

The below list of stretching exercises is what I've been doing for decades. I've picked up different stretching techniques throughout my career as a massage therapist, from a variety of yoga classes, sports training, books, and just watching other people. There are so many different stretch routines and regimens that it would be impossible to cover them all. I've designed this routine to cover the entire body, which addresses balancing all three rings of the torso. It's simple to do, easily transitions from one position to the next, and does not require any equipment.

Stretching is just like everything else in life: the more you do it, the better you'll get. If you're just beginning and feel tight, don't fret. The more you continue with these stretches, the more your tissues will elongate, your joints will open up, and you'll achieve better structural alignment. There is no judgment for how far you can bend. A person who can get their chest to the leg during a hurdle stretch is no better than someone who can't. Bend as far as you comfortably can. Also, there is no need to rush into a given stretch position. Take your time with each one and relax into it. The goal is to become *aware* of the changes that are taking place in your body as you continue to do these stretches over a long period of time (e.g., posture improves, you have fewer aches and pains, walking and/or running becomes easier, etc.).

As a reminder, I've written the number of repetitions or time spent holding a stretch, similar to following a recipe. However, feel free to do more or less, allowing your internal sensations to be your guide.

Deep Breathing

Intent: Lower your heart rate and increase the flow of oxygen into your circulatory system. Loosen your sleeve (limbs) from your core (torso).

This is the same motion as in the warm-up section. Stand with your feet parallel about hip or shoulder width, whichever is widest. Center your body on the floor with your weight balanced through the center of your feet and find the pelvic extension as previously discussed.

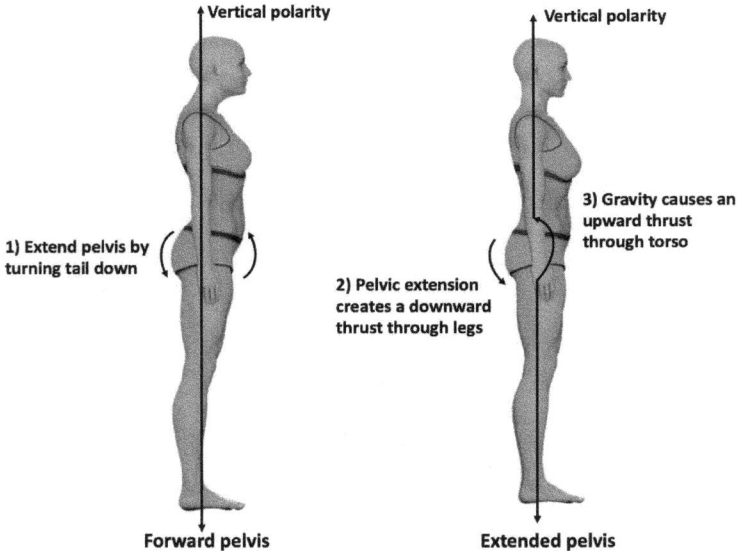

Figure 48: Vertical Polarity

Extend your arms out wide and to the side in a sweeping motion to open the rib cage and raise them above your head while inhaling. Bring your palms face up over your head with your fingers overlapping. Now hold your breath while spreading your elbows out. Imagine someone grabbing both of your elbows and pulling them behind you. Feel your chest expanding. Also, feel free to explore different ranges of motions with this stretch as outlined in the warm-up section under **Deep Breathing**. Repeat three to five times.

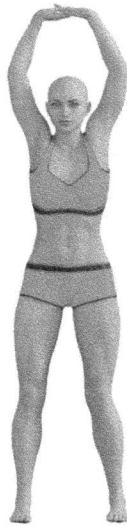

Center

Figure 49: Deep Breathing

Transition to a Squat

Intent: Elongate your spine, stretch your legs, and loosen the rotator muscles of the hips.

Exhaling from your last deep breath, move down into a squat position. Relax and hold the squat position for 30 to 60 seconds or longer. Holding this position is a great way to relax and calm your breathing after a vigorous workout. Your abdominal muscles will be more relaxed due to the support of your legs pushing up on them.

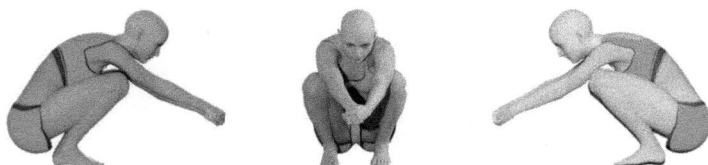

Figure 50: Squat

Hamstring Stretch

Intent: Elongate the hamstring muscles to better balance the pelvic ring.

This is a classic stretch taught pretty much everywhere. Tight hamstrings will pull the pelvis out of alignment. Get down on the floor and into a hurdle position with your right leg out and your left leg to your side, bent at the knee. Be sure to turn your right hip outward so that your foot is pointed up and not out to the side. Lean forward over your right leg as far as is comfortable. Take care not to collapse down from your back. Instead, lean forward, moving from the hips while keeping your back straight over your leg. Be aware of how tight your hamstrings are, and feel the muscles relaxing as you slowly move your chest closer to your leg. If possible, your abdomen should touch your legs first, not your chest.

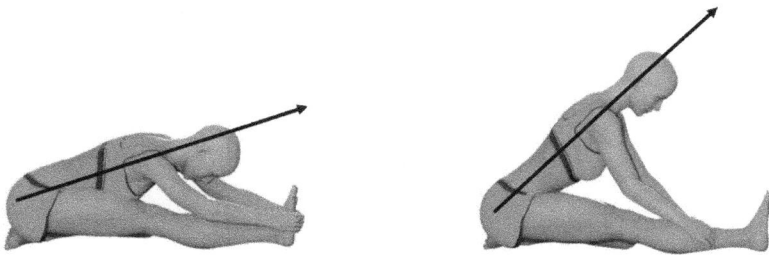

Figure 51: Hamstring Stretch

The takeaway from this stretch is more than just lengthening your hamstrings. Be aware if your leg tends to move farther out to the side as you lean forward. If so, then your hip rotator muscles may be tight and can lead to an unbalanced alignment of the pelvic ring. You may want to hold your leg in place (toes pointed up) with your hands while leaning forward. Holding the joints in place while stretching the connective tissue will better organize the pelvic ring. In turn, this will make your overall gait more balanced and fluid.

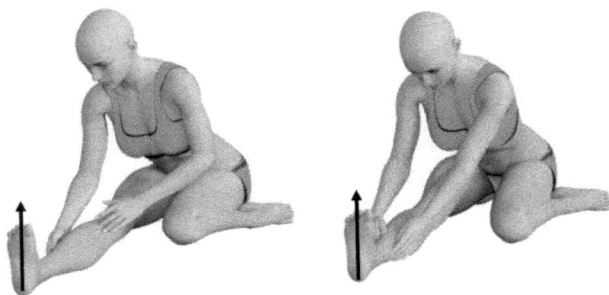

Figure 52: Hamstring Stretch – Toes Up

Hold the hurdle stretch for 90 to 120 seconds to really allow the fascia to elongate. As you hold the stretch, feel free to move your chest closer to your leg. Or stop altogether to straighten your leg if it has turned out and start the stretch again.

Shoulder and Chest Stretch

Intent: Release tension across the chest and open space between the shoulders and chest to better balance the shoulder ring.

While still in the hurdle stretch, place your palms on the floor behind your back and lean back. Slowly shift your weight rhythmically back and forth onto each arm. Feel the stretch across the front of your chest and the inside of your shoulder joints.

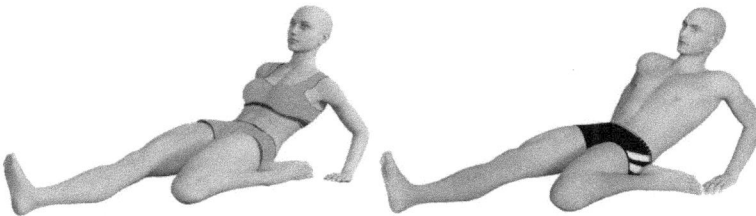

Figure 53: Shoulder and Chest - Lean Back

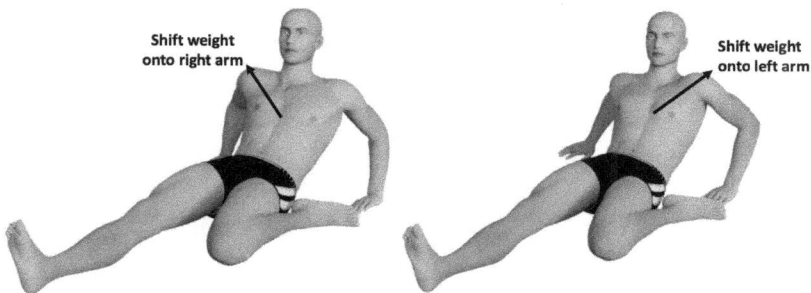

Figure 54: Shoulder and Chest – Shift Weight Side to Side

Inner Core Stretch

Intent: Expand your inner core.

Continue to stay in the hurdle position. Now lie down on your back, bent knee flat on the ground (if you can—don't make it painful), with both arms stretched above your head.

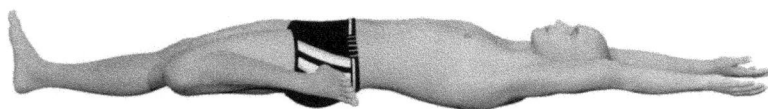

Figure 55: Inner Core Stretch

Inhale by taking a deep breath, raise your chest, and reach with your hand (same side as bent knee) as far as you can while your bent knee is being pulled down in the opposite direction. Imagine the entire side of your body being pulled apart from your core in opposite directions. The arm is extending away from the body and telescoping or reaching, as if you were trying to make it longer. The bent knee is being pulled down by an invisible string and your arm is being pulled up with the sensation that you're being stretched in opposite directions from the middle of your inner core. Feel how this lengthens the tissue in a three-dimensional way through your inner core. Then slowly breathe out and relax your inner core, allowing the body to return to a relaxed starting position.

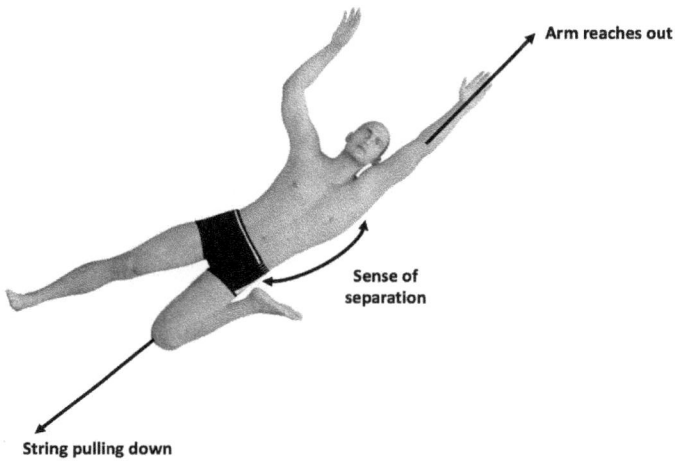

Figure 56: Inner Core – Sense of Separation

Repeat three or four times and move your body with your breath. Breathe slowly. Inhale as you separate the lower half of your body with the upper half. Exhale as you relax back into the starting position.

Switch legs and repeat the hurdle, shoulder/chest, and inner core stretches for the other side of the body.

Butterfly Stretch

Intent: Release the adductor muscles of the leg to better balance the pelvis across the hip joint.

Start in a seated position and bring the soles of your feet together in front of you. Maintain an upright posture in the upper body. Hold your feet with your hands and use your elbows to gently press your knees downward. Focus your intention on the inside of your thighs, in your adductors. Hold this stretch for 60 to 90 seconds.

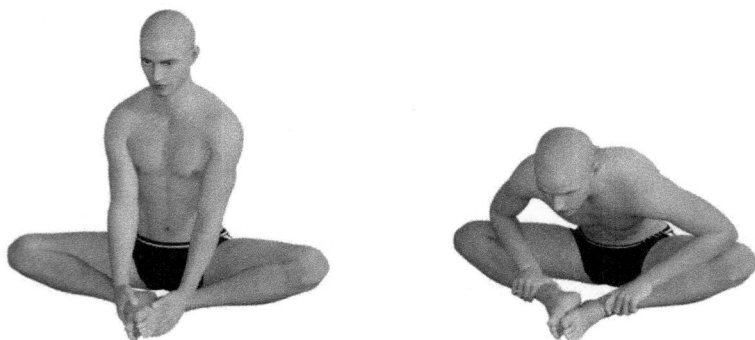

Figure 57: Butterfly Stretch

Glute Stretch

Intent: Loosen the hips and lengthen the round, fleshy parts that form the lower rear area of your pelvis. Allow freer movement across the hip joint and help balance the pelvic ring.

This is also a common stretch. Bring up your right leg (right knee bent) and tuck it under your chest. The left leg is positioned straight back. Roll onto your bent leg and feel the stretch in the gluteus muscles and across the right hip. Hold for 30 to 60 seconds. This stretch is particularly good in reducing discomfort, such as low back pain or tightness in your hips. Switch legs and repeat.

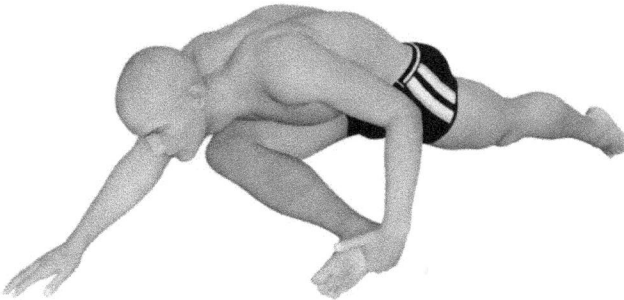

Figure 58: Glute Stretch

Pelvic Lift

Intent: Gain the experience of pelvic extension, which is vital to the overall healthy and efficient structural integration of the body.

Lie on your back again and bend your knees while your feet remain on the floor. Keep your feet parallel to each other. This is a two-step process. First, turn the pelvis in ("tail under") and allow the sacral hinge to lengthen the spine. Next, push into the floor with your heels, which will extend your knees forward, lifting the pelvis off the floor. Keep your abdomen relaxed and allow the spine to hang back from the knees. There shouldn't be any tension between the pelvis and thighs and/or hamstrings. The work comes from pushing the heels into the ground. You're giving your body the experience of the integrated relationship between the pelvis and the lumbar spine by not allowing extraneous muscle groups to engage, which can unbalance the pelvic ring.

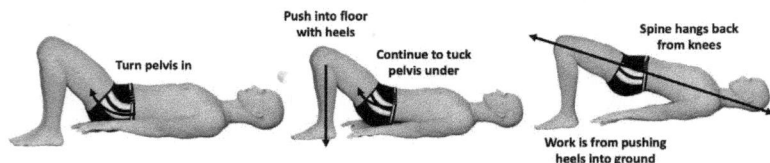

Figure 59: Pelvic Lift

Back Roll

Intent: Lengthen the back as well as reinforce a unified sense of the lumbar spine and core.

Start in a seated position with your back upward, then bring your knees up to your chest with hands clasped in front of the knees to hold them in place. Begin by shifting your weight back and rolling backward onto your shoulders. Then shift your weight forward to roll up onto your pelvis, almost back into the starting sitting position, and then roll back again. Continue to roll back and forth, getting a sense of your spine lengthening as it presses against the ground.

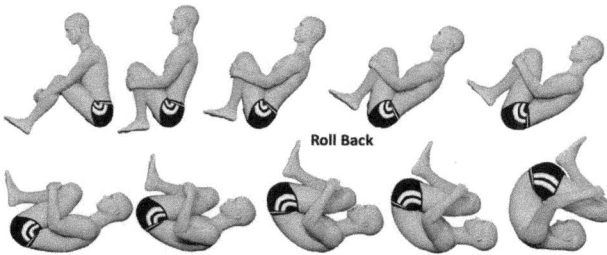

Figure 60: Back Roll – Rock Back

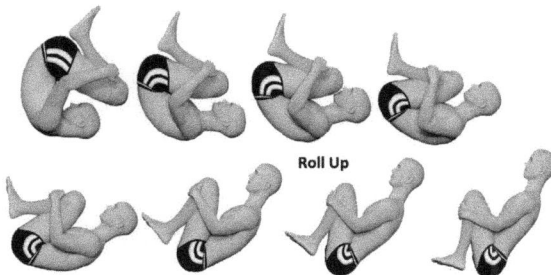

Figure 61: Back Roll – Rock Forward

Feel free to play with different speeds, rocking faster or slower to further gain a unified sense of the lumbar spine and core. Also, play around with rolling off the spine by slightly shifting your weight either to the right or left.

Back Roll (Ankles Overhead) Stretch

Intent: Maintain an integrated stretch across multiple joints at the same time, to build balance within your core.

This is a multifaceted stretch that may be a little more advanced than most people are willing to do. Don't worry if you can't get it completely. Do as much as you can and work on it. You should feel the stretch across your chest, shoulders, back, arms, neck, and pelvis.

While doing the back rolls, roll onto your back and lift your legs, then extend them straight out over and behind your head. Allow your toes to rest on the floor behind your head and straighten out both legs by locking your knees.

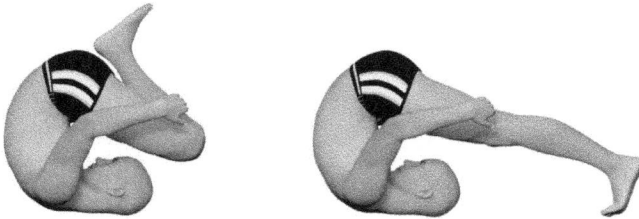

Figure 62: Back Roll (Ankles Overhead)

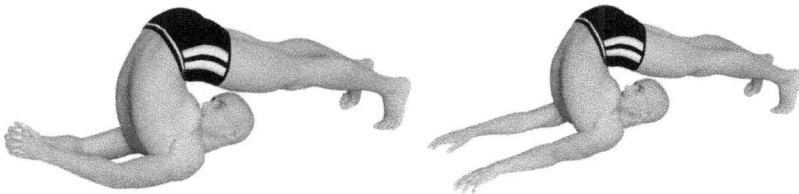

Figure 63: Hands Clasped behind Back – Hands on Floor

Next, grasp your fingers together behind your back. If you need to, walk up with your shoulders so you can get your arms closer to each other behind your back. Comfortably clasp your fingers together while pressing the palms of your hands together and lock your elbows. If that's too much of a strain, leave your hands unclasped on the floor behind your head.

Hold for 30 to 60 seconds. Be sure to breathe normally as this position can put pressure on your diaphragm. This stretch will help to build balance within your core.

Abdominal Balancing

Intent: Strengthen your core while maintaining balance.

Push your legs out and lift the torso again, and as you return the legs to the floor, pause halfway. Hold your arms out for balance. Hold the position for 30 to 60 seconds.

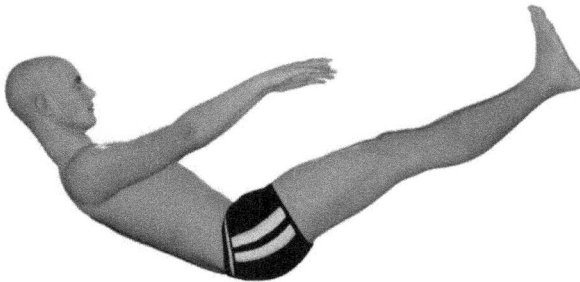

Figure 64: Abdominal Balancing

Double Hamstring Stretch

Intent: Elongate the hamstring muscles and allow a more balanced integration of the pelvic ring.

This is the same as the hamstring stretch described earlier, except you're stretching the hamstrings of both legs simultaneously.

Extend your legs forward and straighten them. If your feet are falling to the sides, you can grab each leg with your hands to turn your hips inward so that your feet stay pointed up. This will help to eliminate hip turnout, which is a large source of unbalanced movement of the pelvic ring.

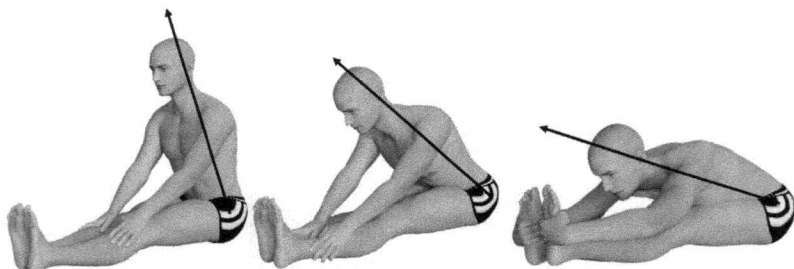

Figure 65: Double Hamstring Stretch

Reach your hands as far as you can comfortably and place them on your legs. This could be under or over the calf, around the ankle or possibly on the bottom of your foot. Don't worry about how far you can bend down. It's more important to keep your back straight and not collapse it. Lean forward rather than pulling yourself down. You want to build awareness of how tight your hamstrings are and feel the muscles relaxing as you slowly move your chest closer to your legs. Hold the stretch for 90 to 120 seconds to really allow the fascia to elongate. As you hold the stretch, feel free to move your chest closer to your legs. Or stop altogether to straighten your legs if they have turned out and start the stretch again.

Lower Leg Stretch

Intent: Release the muscles and organize the lower legs, ankles, and knees to better align. Organizing the legs also releases length up the back.

Grab the backs of your toes with each hand to stretch the soleus and popliteus muscles. Hold the stretch for 60 to 90 seconds.

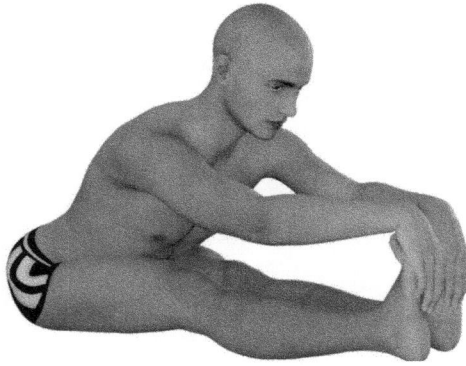

Figure 66: Lower Leg Stretch

Lunge Stretch

Intent: Open the hip joints to better organize the pelvic ring.

This stretch will release core muscles like the iliopsoas and other sleeve muscles such as the glutes, hamstrings, quads, and even muscles in the ankles, which will lead to greater organization of the pelvic ring.

There are many different types of lunges, including but not limited to the forward lunge, reverse lunge, lateral lunge, curtsy lunge, and lunge with rotation. Feel free to explore these lunges, but I'm just going to list one type: the lunge elbow to instep.

Start by bringing the right leg up into a lunge position with the left knee on the floor and the ankle behind. Place your left hand on the floor even with your right foot. Then place your right elbow on the floor adjacent to the right knee. Gently push your weight forward and hold this position for 30 seconds. Repeat for the other side.

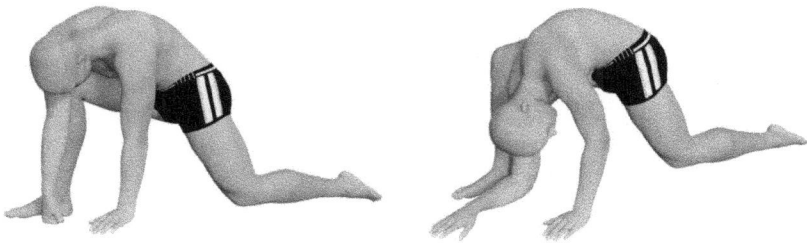

Figure 67: Lunge Stretch

Middle Splits

Intent: Structurally align the pelvis across the hip joint.

This stretch releases the adductor muscles of the leg as well as the attachments on the pelvis. Tight adductors will twist the pelvis out of alignment. The stretch will also reduce hip turnout, improving balance in the legs and the pelvic ring.

Start by sitting down and spreading your feet as wide apart from each other as you can. Be sure that your toes are pointed up. Spread your feet away from each other as the tension slowly releases by further pushing your legs out. Put your hands on the ground in front of you for support.

Go as far as you can comfortably, keep your arms extended, and hold the position. If you can go farther, drop down onto your forearms and lean forward to increase the tension in your groin area. Hold the position for roughly 30 seconds. Then spread your feet farther apart again by pushing your legs out. Lean forward again and hold the position, feeling the tension in the groin area, for an additional 60 to 90 seconds.

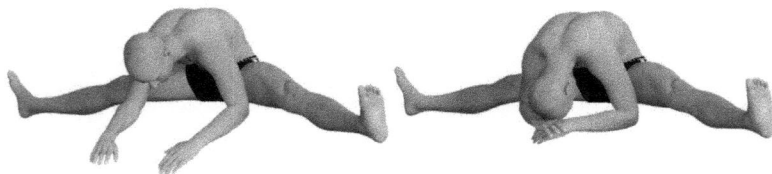

Figure 68: Middle Splits

Lumbar Spine Twist

Intent: Organize the core.

In this case, the core we are organizing is a webwork of connections beginning with the inner thigh, which releases the pelvis, through the lumbar spine and up to the diaphragm ring. This stretch should leave you with an open balance from feet to diaphragm.

Lying flat on your back, cross one leg over the other by putting one foot under the knee of the other leg and twisting your hips and spine while twisting your head in the opposite direction. Keep your opposite arm outstretched. Approach the stretch gently. Do not force yourself into the position. You can hold on to your bent knee to make the stretch stronger. Use your breath to move deeper into the stretch and hold for roughly 60 seconds.

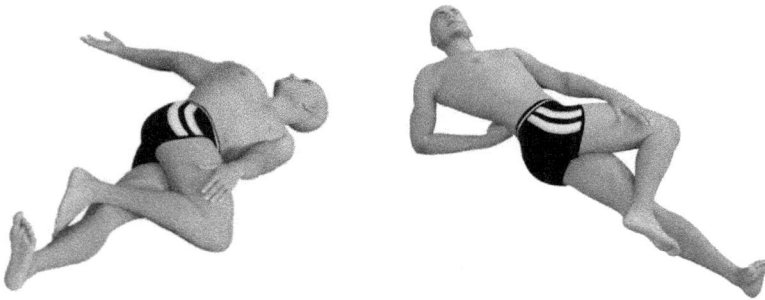

Figure 69: Lumbar Spine Twist

Cobra Stretch

Intent: Lengthen the lumbar spine while releasing tension in your abdomen.

This is another good motion to structurally balance your core. Tight abdominals will pull your rib cage down, tilting your diaphragm ring and causing your shoulders to slouch and slump.

Start by lying flat on your stomach. Point your toes behind you and place your hands under your shoulders. Keep your elbows close to your ribs. Press your palms into the floor as you lift your chest off the ground. Slightly bend your elbows and hug them to your sides. Hold this position for 30 seconds.

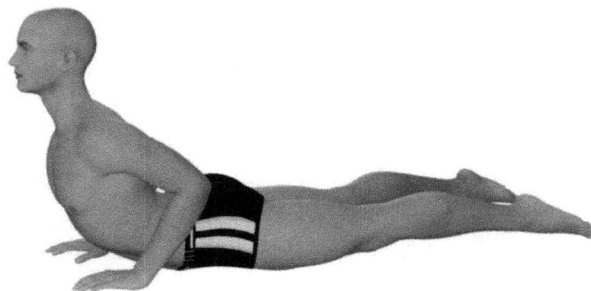

Figure 70: Cobra Stretch

Cat–Cow Stretch

Intent: Improve the structural integration of your whole body along the central axis of the core.

This stretch activates the tailbone and releases tension in the neck and upper back. It also improves the organization of the neck, shoulders, spine, and pelvis.

Beginning with the cat pose, start on your hands and knees, aligning your wrists underneath your shoulders and your knees underneath your hips. Extend your neck by looking up and out, and tilt your pelvis back so your tailbone sticks up.

Move into cow pose by exhaling and tipping your pelvis forward, tucking your tailbone, and allowing this movement to transmit the energy through your spine. Your spine will naturally round. Draw your navel toward your spine and lower your head.

Move back into cat pose by inhaling and tilting your pelvis back, sticking up your tailbone. Again, allow the movement to transmit the energy through your spine. The spine will naturally arch as the head gently rises. Repeat the cat–cow stretch on each inhale and exhale, matching the movement to your own breath. Continue for five to ten breaths, moving the whole spine.

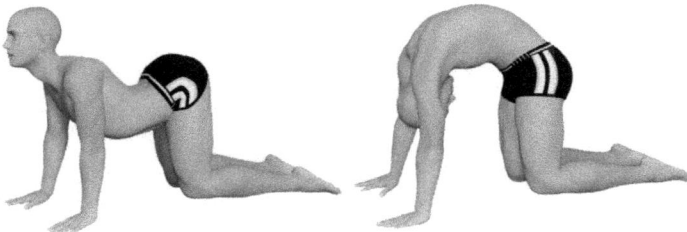

Figure 71: Cat–Cow Stretch

Backward Palm Lock with Head and Neck Rolls

Intent: Finish up the integration of your core with the head and neck.

Lean back and sit down on your ankles. This movement is a repeat of the one described in the warm-up section, except now you're sitting on your ankles instead of standing. Hold the stretch for 30 to 60 seconds.

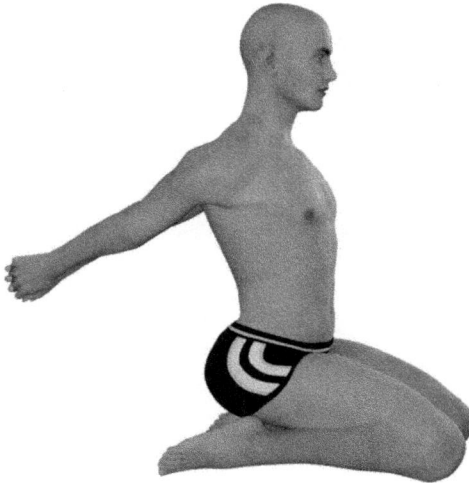

Figure 72: Backward Palm Lock with Head and Neck Rolls

Congratulations! You're good for another 24 hours.

CHAPTER 8

DEVELOP YOUR PERSONAL WEEKLY WORKOUT PLAN

B y now you understand why exercise is fundamental to building greater awareness of your body using the concepts of expansional balance. You know how to incorporate expansional balance into your exercise regimen with the intent of moving with no resistance in the joints. And you're aware of how important it is to bring the three rings of the torso into a parallel relationship with each other to improve the structural organization of your core and sleeve.

You've also learned how the exercises in this book will release contracted fascia and bring awareness of aberrant holding patterns and compensatory movements. These exercises will aid in releasing tension and opening the joints so they can move more freely and fluidly. An integrated feeling of the whole body can be attained. You also hopefully understand how to develop the willpower to exercise and make it a daily part of your life.

Ready to improve your quality of life? Then let's discuss how much exercise you want to do and develop a custom workout plan that's right for you. Your plan can obviously change over time according to your goals, current level of physical condition, and what feels right. Now, let's begin to build your personal workout plan step-by-step.

Step 1: Determine how much time you're willing to commit

If you're going to be successful at making exercise a daily activity, then the first step is to *determine how much time you are willing to spend.* This is crucial. Your greatest challenge to developing a regular workout practice is determining the amount of time you'll commit to. Exercising is the easy part.

Most importantly, the amount of time you determine is non-negotiable, either with others or yourself. When it's time to exercise, then that becomes your highest priority. Don't allow outside events or other people to interrupt you. If need be, tell others that you have blocked out time to do your workout and you are not to be disturbed. Clearly, if you're ill or a crisis arises, then that situation will need to take priority over your workout, but otherwise this time is yours and no one else's.

Step 2: Input your time into my exercise routine formula

Once you have decided how much time to commit, the second step is to decide on the proper exercise formula. Let's say you've blocked out an hour each day for five days a week. (We'll call this the *day time period*.) Your workout plan would be to distribute all three types of exercises equally within this hour: 20 minutes a day for endurance, 20 minutes a day for strength, and 20 minutes a day for flexibility. The formula would look like this:

20S/20E/20F = 1 hour/day for 5 days/week

As you get stronger and more flexible and build up endurance, you can bump it up to 30 minutes a day for strength, 30 minutes a day for endurance, and 30 minutes a day for flexibility. Then your workout plan formula would look like this:

30S/30E/30F = 1.5 hours/day for 5 days/week

Say you want to concentrate more on cardio and less on strength exercises during that hour and a half per day? Then alter your formula to:

20S/45E/25F = 1.5 hours/day for 5 days/week

It doesn't have to be the same amount of time every day either. It's good to mix it up to keep things interesting. Feel free to spread your formula out if your schedule permits. If some days you can't get the time, or simply want shorter day time periods, then break out your day time periods into separate formulas. Using the example above, say you want to concentrate on cardio only three days per week while increasing your day time period on flexibility exercises for two days per week; then your formula would be:

20S/45E/25F = 1.5 hours/day for 3 days/week
15S/0E/45F = 1 hour/day for 2 days/week

Here's another example. If you want to concentrate on strength exercises three days per week and concentrate on cardio and flexibility for the other two, then the formula would be:

45S/10E/5F = 1 hour/day for 3 days/week
0S/45E/45F = 1.5 hours/day for 2 days/week

Try not to overcomplicate this process. I've listed only five examples of exercise routine formulas, but there is an infinite number of combinations to choose from. As your body gains greater awareness, you'll want to modify your exercise routine formula to adjust to what feels right for you. The key is to determine how much time per day you're willing to commit to and then input that time into your personal exercise formula.

Step 3: Write down the exercise formula into a weekly plan

The last step is to write down a weekly schedule for strength, endurance, and flexibility per your individualized exercise formula(s). Populate your times into the weekly schedule using the exercises I've described in this book. Let's use the 30S/30E/30F example from the previous section. Your weekly plan would look like this.

Table 1: Weekly Strength Plan Example (30 Minutes)

	Strength	Monday	Tuesday	Wednesday	Thursday	Friday
UPPER BODY	Chest Press/Incline Press	x				x
	Overhead Press		x		x	
	Pull-Back		x		x	
	Lateral Raise	x				x
	Pull-Down/Chin-Up	x				x
	Pectoral Fly		x		x	
	Rear Deltoid Fly		x		x	
	Dip	x				x
ABDOMINAL	Stomach Crunch			x		x
	Rotating Sit-Up			x		x
	Leg Lift			x		x
	Side Bend					x
	Back Extension			x		x
ARMS	Biceps Curl	x		x		
	Triceps Curl	x		x		
	Forearm Curl	x		x		
LEGS	Leg Extension		x		x	
	Leg Curl		x		x	
	Leg Press (Squat)	x		x		
	Calf Extension	x		x		
	Hip Adduction		x		x	
	Hip Abduction		x		x	

The strength routines I've listed (described earlier) are designed to complete a full-body workout that engages all skeletal muscles and joints of the body. A complete circuit (all combined exercises for one day) should take approximately 25 to 30 minutes. The exercises are done for 10 to 12 repetitions per set for three sets each with approximately 30 seconds between each set.

Whatever level of intensity you choose, always use enough weight so that the last rep of the last set is a bit of a struggle, but not such a struggle that you're making compensatory movements with some part of your body not intended for the specific exercise.

Table 2: Weekly Cardio Plan Example (30 Minutes)

Endurance	Monday	Tuesday	Wednesday	Thursday	Friday
Brisk Walking	30 MIN	30 MIN	30 MIN	30 MIN	30 MIN
Jogging/Running/ Sprinting	30 MIN	30 MIN	30 MIN	30 MIN	30 MIN
Bicycling/ Stationary Bike	30 MIN	30 MIN	30 MIN	30 MIN	30 MIN

You can choose from brisk walking, jogging, running, cycling, a combination of each, or any cardio workout that increases your heart rate for a sustained period of 30 minutes. Whatever workout you choose, I recommend that you maintain an increased heart rate that causes you to break out into a sweat. Work out till you're tired at the end. No need to push beyond that. The more cardio exercises you do over time, the longer it will take to make yourself tired. This in turn means you may want to eventually lengthen your workout sessions.

Table 3: Weekly Stretch Plan Example (30 Minutes)

Flexibility	Monday	Tuesday	Wednesday	Thursday	Friday
Deep Breathing	x	x	x	x	x
Squat	x	x	x	x	x
Hamstring Stretch	x	x	x	x	x
Shoulder and Chest Stretch	x	x	x	x	x
Inner Core Stretch	x	x	x	x	x
Butterfly Stretch	x	x	x	x	x
Glute Stretch	x	x	x	x	x
Pelvic Lift	x	x	x	x	x
Back Roll	x	x	x	x	x
Back Roll (Ankles Overhead) Stretch	x	x	x	x	x
Abdominal Balancing	x	x	x	x	x
Double Hamstring Stretch	x	x	x	x	x
Lower Leg Stretch	x	x	x	x	x
Lunge Stretch	x	x	x	x	x
Middle Splits	x	x	x	x	x
Lumbar Spine Twist	x	x	x	x	x
Cobra Stretch	x	x	x	x	x
Cat–Cow Stretch	x	x	x	x	x
Backward Palm Lock with Head and Neck Rolls	x	x	x	x	x

The stretch routines I've designed cover the entire body and address balancing all three rings of the torso. It should take approximately 30 minutes to complete all of them depending on the time you hold each stretch. Take notice of the changes that are taking place in your body as you continue to do these stretches over a long period of time (e.g., posture improves, you have fewer aches and pains, walking and/ or running becomes easier, etc.).

Step 4: Execute your plan

Now comes the easy part. You've set aside time, you've created your exercise routine formula, and your workout plan is solid. Now you need to execute the plan. Remember, how you execute the plan depends entirely on your current level of fitness. Don't worry about pushing yourself. What's important is that you do the exercises in your plan repetitively. You will continue to get stronger, build endurance, and become more flexible over time. Some days will be easier than others, but if you stick with it, you'll see the results.

CHAPTER 9

EXAMPLE WORKOUT PLANS

Keep in mind that these exercise plans are just examples and won't fit everyone. It's important to be aware of your current level of fitness and not attempt to take on too much or too little. It will take weeks, or months, of experimenting with different exercises and schedules to develop a workout plan that is right for you. Moreover, you don't have to follow the same workout plan every week. Feel free to have multiple plans that you can switch out weekly or monthly depending on how you're feeling. The best approach is to be flexible and remember that there is no perfect workout program for everyone.

Table 4: 30S/30E/30F Weekly Workout Plan

30S / 30E / 30F						
	Strength	**Monday**	**Tuesday**	**Wednesday**	**Thursday**	**Friday**
UPPER BODY	Chest Press/ Incline Press	x				x
	Overhead Press		x		x	
	Pull-Back		x		x	
	Lateral Raise	x				x
	Pull-Down/Chin-Up	x				x
	Pectoral Fly		x		x	
	Rear Deltoid Fly		x		x	
	Dip	x				x
ABDOMINAL	Stomach Crunch			x		x
	Rotating Sit-Up			x		x
	Leg Lift			x		x
	Side Bend					x
	Back Extension			x		x
ARMS	Biceps Curl	x		x		
	Triceps Curl	x		x		
	Forearm Curl	x		x		
LEGS	Leg Extension		x		x	
	Leg Curl		x		x	
	Leg Press (Squat)	x		x		
	Calf Extension	x		x		
	Hip Adduction		x		x	
	Hip Abduction		x		x	

Endurance	**Monday**	**Tuesday**	**Wednesday**	**Thursday**	**Friday**
Brisk Walking					
Jogging/Running/ Sprinting	30 MIN		30 MIN		30 MIN
Bicycling/ Stationary Bike		30 MIN		30 MIN	

Flexibility	Monday	Tuesday	Wednesday	Thursday	Friday
Deep Breathing	x	x	x	x	x
Squat	x	x	x	x	x
Hamstring Stretch	x	x	x	x	x
Shoulder and Chest Stretch	x	x	x	x	x
Inner Core Stretch	x	x	x	x	x
Butterfly Stretch	x	x	x	x	x
Glute Stretch	x	x	x	x	x
Pelvic Lift	x	x	x	x	x
Back Roll	x	x	x	x	x
Back Roll (Ankles Overhead) Stretch	x	x	x	x	x
Abdominal Balancing	x	x	x	x	x
Double Hamstring Stretch	x	x	x	x	x
Lower Leg Stretch	x	x	x	x	x
Lunge Stretch	x	x	x	x	x
Middle Splits	x	x	x	x	x
Lumbar Spine Twist	x	x	x	x	x
Cobra Stretch	x	x	x	x	x
Cat–Cow Stretch	x	x	x	x	x
Backward Palm Lock with Head and Neck Rolls	x	x	x	x	x

Table 5: 20S/20E/20F Weekly Workout Plan

20S / 20E / 20F						
Strength		**Monday**	**Tuesday**	**Wednesday**	**Thursday**	**Friday**
UPPER BODY	Chest Press/ Incline Press	x				x
	Overhead Press				x	
	Pull-Back				x	
	Lateral Raise		x			
	Pull-Down/Chin-Up	x				x
	Pectoral Fly		x		x	
	Rear Deltoid Fly		x		x	
	Dip	x				x
ABDOMINAL	Stomach Crunch			x		x
	Rotating Sit-Up					x
	Leg Lift			x		
	Side Bend			x		
	Back Extension					x
ARMS	Biceps Curl	x		x		
	Triceps Curl		x			
	Forearm Curl		x			
LEGS	Leg Extension		x		x	
	Leg Curl		x		x	
	Leg Press (Squat)	x		x		
	Calf Extension	x		x		

Endurance	**Monday**	**Tuesday**	**Wednesday**	**Thursday**	**Friday**
Brisk Walking					
Jogging/Running/ Sprinting	20 MIN		20 MIN		20 MIN
Bicycling/ Stationary Bike		20 MIN		20 MIN	

Flexibility	Monday	Tuesday	Wednesday	Thursday	Friday
Deep Breathing	x	x	x	x	x
Squat	x	x	x	x	x
Hamstring Stretch	x	x	x	x	x
Shoulder and Chest Stretch	x	x	x	x	x
Inner Core Stretch	x	x	x	x	x
Butterfly Stretch	x	x	x	x	x
Glute Stretch	x	x	x	x	x
Lunge Stretch	x	x	x	x	x
Middle Splits	x	x	x	x	x
Lumbar Spine Twist	x	x	x	x	x
Cobra Stretch	x	x	x	x	x
Backward Palm Lock with Head and Neck Rolls	x	x	x	x	x

Table 6: 20S/45E/25F Weekly Workout Plan

20S / 45E / 25F						
Strength		**Monday**	**Tuesday**	**Wednesday**	**Thursday**	**Friday**
UPPER BODY	Chest Press/ Incline Press	x				x
	Overhead Press				x	
	Pull-Back				x	
	Lateral Raise		x			
	Pull-Down/Chin-Up	x				x
	Pectoral Fly		x		x	
	Rear Deltoid Fly		x		x	
	Dip	x				x
ABDOMINAL	Stomach Crunch			x		x
	Rotating Sit-Up					x
	Leg Lift			x		
	Side Bend			x		
	Back Extension					x
ARMS	Biceps Curl	x		x		
	Triceps Curl		x			
	Forearm Curl		x			
LEGS	Leg Extension		x		x	
	Leg Curl		x		x	
	Leg Press (Squat)	x		x		
	Calf Extension	x		x		

Endurance	**Monday**	**Tuesday**	**Wednesday**	**Thursday**	**Friday**
Brisk Walking					
Jogging/Running/ Sprinting	15 MIN	15 MIN	15 MIN	15 MIN	15 MIN
Bicycling/ Stationary Bike	30 MIN	30 MIN	30 MIN	30 MIN	30 MIN

Flexibility	Monday	Tuesday	Wednesday	Thursday	Friday
Deep Breathing	x	x	x	x	x
Squat	x	x	x	x	x
Hamstring Stretch	x	x	x	x	x
Shoulder and Chest Stretch	x	x	x	x	x
Inner Core Stretch	x	x	x	x	x
Butterfly Stretch	x	x	x	x	x
Glute Stretch	x	x	x	x	x
Back Roll	x	x	x	x	x
Double Hamstring Stretch	x	x	x	x	x
Lunge Stretch	x	x	x	x	x
Middle Splits	x	x	x	x	x
Lumbar Spine Twist	x	x	x	x	x
Cobra Stretch	x	x	x	x	x
Backward Palm Lock with Head and Neck Rolls	x	x	x	x	x

Table 7: 20S/45E/25F – 15S/0E/45F Weekly Workout Plan

20S / 45E / 25F – 15S / 0E / 45F						
	Strength	**Monday**	**Tuesday**	**Wednesday**	**Thursday**	**Friday**
UPPER BODY	Chest Press/ Incline Press	x		x		
	Overhead Press				x	
	Pull-Back				x	
	Lateral Raise	x				
	Pull-Down/Chin-Up	x		x		
	Pectoral Fly	x				
	Rear Deltoid Fly			x		
	Dip	x				x
ABDOMINAL	Stomach Crunch			x		x
	Rotating Sit-Up					x
	Leg Lift			x		
	Side Bend			x		
	Back Extension					x
ARMS	Biceps Curl	x				x
	Triceps Curl		x			x
	Forearm Curl		x			
LEGS	Leg Extension				x	
	Leg Curl				x	
	Leg Press (Squat)		x			
	Calf Extension		x			

Endurance	**Monday**	**Tuesday**	**Wednesday**	**Thursday**	**Friday**
Brisk Walking					
Jogging/Running/ Sprinting					
Bicycling/ Stationary Bike	45 MIN		45 MIN		45 MIN

Flexibility	Monday	Tuesday	Wednesday	Thursday	Friday
Deep Breathing	x	x	x	x	x
Squat		x		x	
Hamstring Stretch	x	x	x	x	x
Shoulder and Chest Stretch	x	x	x	x	x
Inner Core Stretch	x	x	x	x	x
Butterfly Stretch	x	x	x	x	x
Glute Stretch	x	x	x	x	x
Pelvic Lift		x		x	
Back Roll		x		x	
Back Roll (Ankles Overhead) Stretch		x		x	
Double Hamstring Stretch	x	x	x	x	x
Lower Leg Stretch		x			x
Lunge Stretch	x	x	x	x	x
Middle Splits	x	x	x	x	x
Lumbar Spine Twist	x	x	x	x	x
Cobra Stretch	x	x	x	x	x
Cat–Cow Stretch		x			x
Backward Palm Lock with Head and Neck Rolls	x	x	x	x	x

Table 8: 45S/10E/5F – 0S/45E/45F Weekly Workout Plan

45S / 10E / 5F – 0S / 45E / 45F						
Strength		**Monday**	**Tuesday**	**Wednesday**	**Thursday**	**Friday**
UPPER BODY	Chest Press/ Incline Press	x				x
	Overhead Press	x		x		
	Pull-Back			x		x
	Lateral Raise	x				x
	Pull-Down/Chin-Up	x				x
	Pectoral Fly	x				x
	Rear Deltoid Fly	x				x
	Dip	x				x
ABDOMINAL	Stomach Crunch			x		x
	Rotating Sit-Up			x		x
	Leg Lift			x		x
	Side Bend			x		x
	Back Extension			x		x
ARMS	Biceps Curl	x		x		
	Triceps Curl	x		x		
	Forearm Curl	x		x		
LEGS	Leg Extension	x		x		
	Leg Curl	x		x		
	Leg Press (Squat)	x		x		
	Calf Extension	x		x		
	Hip Adduction					x
	Hip Abduction					x

Endurance	**Monday**	**Tuesday**	**Wednesday**	**Thursday**	**Friday**
Brisk Walking	10 MIN		10 MIN		10 MIN
Jogging/Running/ Sprinting		45 MIN		45 MIN	
Bicycling/ Stationary Bike					

Flexibility	Monday	Tuesday	Wednesday	Thursday	Friday
Deep Breathing	x	x	x	x	x
Squat		x		x	
Hamstring Stretch	x	x	x	x	x
Shoulder and Chest Stretch		x		x	
Inner Core Stretch	x	x	x	x	x
Butterfly Stretch		x		x	
Glute Stretch		x		x	
Pelvic Lift		x		x	
Back Roll		x		x	
Back Roll (Ankles Overhead) Stretch		x		x	
Double Hamstring Stretch		x		x	
Lower Leg Stretch		x		x	
Lunge Stretch		x		x	
Middle Splits		x		x	
Lumbar Spine Twist		x		x	
Cobra Stretch		x		x	
Cat–Cow Stretch		x		x	
Backward Palm Lock with Head and Neck Rolls	x	x	x	x	x

CHAPTER 10

EXERCISE FOR A HIGHER QUALITY OF LIFE

The workout regimen I have described in this book is a means to a higher quality of life. Each exercise in this book is a building block that will help bring you closer to understanding your body and how it moves in the field of gravity. Hopefully you understand by now why each exercise is important, what the intent of each exercise is, and how it relates to the concept of expansional balance. Together, these strength, endurance, and flexibility exercises create a more holistic approach to health and fitness as opposed to maximizing performance to compete with others.

I want to close with a few reminders that will help you be successful with your own expansional balance exercise regimen.

1. Move with Awareness

While performing any exercise, whether in your own workout routine or the ones described in this book, awareness is key. Moving with awareness will help you recognize aberrant holding patterns and compensatory movements so you can develop healthier movement patterns.

This is not always easy to do alone, however. One remedy is to seek out a professional to aid in raising your body awareness. Sessions with a massage therapist can help restore some of your lost body awareness and even correct some of the negative conditions that are causing pain and discomfort. I would, however, caution you to not become dependent on a therapist's hands to facilitate the results of a regimental workout done with awareness. Moreover, it can get expensive to visit a therapist regularly.

Instead, focus on building your own capacity for self-awareness when doing these exercises, and you'll be developing an invaluable skill that will serve you forever.

2. Exercise Regularly

A successful workout regimen involves performing exercises at the right intensity and for the appropriate amount of time. It also requires consistency, and it's here where many people fall short. A little exercise is always better than none, but to truly live a healthy life you'll need the will to make your workout routine a regular part of your lifestyle. Make your workout a habit, as opposed to disciplined behavior or a means of achieving a goal. Regular vigorous exercise is just something that must become a habit to maintain a healthy level of strength, endurance, and flexibility. The alternative is to become weak, sluggish, and stiff.

3. Customize If You Need To

In this book I've detailed an exercise regimen that helps to reorganize your body in a more efficient and neutral alignment through a regimented workout that engages all muscles of the body. It's a full-body workout for a reason: only doing some exercises and neglecting others can lead to weakness in one part of the body while creating a pattern of overcompensation in another.

What if the exercises in this book aren't working for you? Thankfully, the concept of expansional balance can be incorporated into any workout. There are many different types of exercise regimens and intensity levels to choose from, depending on your ability and goals. Incorporating the concept of expansional balance into your own workout regimen can make your workouts more interesting, and more likely that you'll stick with exercising in the long run.

A Higher Quality of Life

I hope what you've learned in this book will help you feel stronger, more energetic and mentally alert, and free of aches and pains. By incorporating the concepts of expansional balance and how it relates to the three rings of the torso into a vigorous exercise regimen like the one in this book, you'll be able to enjoy more of your life thanks to your ability to move pain free, with greater strength, endurance, and flexibility.

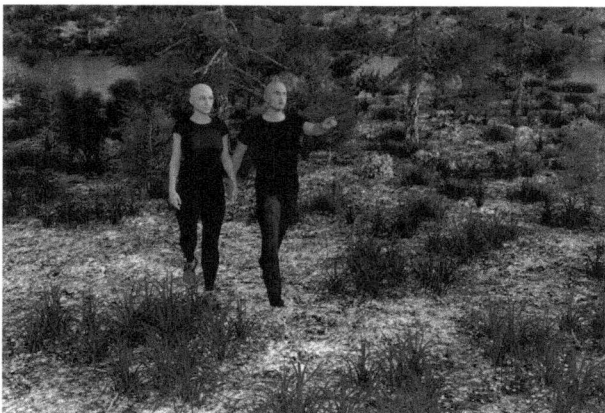

Figure 73: Higher Quality of Life

ACKNOWLEDGMENTS

I want to thank Ed Maupin for being an amazing teacher, mentor, and friend. I have fond memories working and laughing with him. Ed taught me the concepts of Structural Integration and its relationship to expansional balance. Ed's instructions on the ten-session series of Structural Integration were not only invaluable in my practice, but also in my personal growth as a massage therapist.

My stepfather John Armitage started to teach me how to exercise when I was nine years old. Whether circuit training in the basement or kicking the soccer ball back and forth to each other while running in the backyard, he taught me the importance of maintaining a strong, healthy body.

Last but not least, my loving wife, Julie Dougan, who encouraged me to write this book. I am grateful for her patience and support.

ABOUT THE AUTHOR

Brian started out his career path as a massage therapist in the late '80s. After a ten-year stint he switched careers to work as an engineer for a large defense contractor. Eventually retiring from the defense industry, he now owns a small real estate investment company. Brian has B.A. degrees in physics and astronomy from Northern Arizona University and a master's in business administration (MBA) from the University of Arizona, and is a Holistic Health Practitioner (HHP) with over 1,000 hours of training in massage and somatic practices from the International Professional School of Bodywork (IPSB) in San Diego, CA.

During the late '80s, Brian studied and practiced a method of bodywork called Structural Integration. Since then, he has studied, interned, taught, and practiced Structural Integration for many decades. Brian has also been exercising at fitness centers regularly since the age of 18. He has unique insights based on his own personal experiences dealing with the fitness and the holistic health industries. Over the course of decades, he has learned to use the concepts of Structural Integration in his own exercise regimen, which he calls Expansional Balance.

Brian currently lives in Tucson, AZ with his wife Julie. You can friend Brian on his Facebook page Expansional Balance; visit his website and leave a review at expansionalbalancebook.com; or write to him at briandougan@expansionalbalancebook.com.

INDEX